Gut Health

Stop Wasting Your Time on Trying to Have a Healthier Gut

(Healing Herbs & Clean Eating Guide for Optimal Digestive Health)

Ronald Payne

I0095429

Published By **Phil Dawson**

Ronald Payne

Gut Health: Stop Wasting Your Time on Trying to Have a Healthier Gut (Healing Herbs & Clean Eating Guide for Optimal Digestive Health)

ISBN 978-1-998769-18-6

Legal & Disclaimer

TABLE OF CONTENTS

Chapter 1: What Is Gut Health?

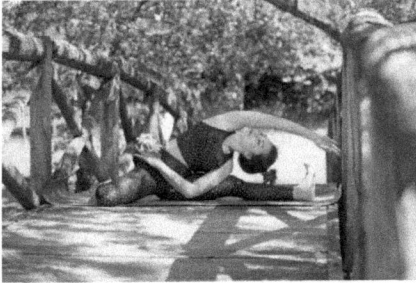

Let's discuss your Gut's function and how it works!

To know more about Gut Health it is essential to be aware of the Gut and how it works within the body of a human. Gut is it is a Canal or tube through which food gets processed and circulates. It's a route for food particles from the mouth to the anus.

In this way, Gut helps the food by moving and mixing juices, and also to provide minerals, vitamins, nutrients and electrolytes essential to our daily lives while protecting our body from harmful materials.

Microbiota or flora determines your Gut Health. In your digestive tract 40 trillion chemists working hard to help to digest your meals creating essential nutrients you cannot make by yourself, protecting yourself from diseases and even determining what elements of your DNA are manifest and which are inactive.

The amazing creatures are fungiand bacteria and other single-celled creatures. They're a bigger aspect of your identity than you've thought of!

There is a 10x increase in bacteria found in the gut in comparison to the rest of the body. The health of your gut is compromised when there is a lack of balance in the amount and diversity of the bacteria that reside in your gut. Healthy old age is a sign of your healthy bacteria , or good gut health.

Gut plays a role in the process of metabolism. For a healthy metabolism we must make sure that the gut flora balances and is diverse. This is why we should be concerned about the following aspects:

* Nutrition

* Probiotic foods can be used to aid in digestion.

* Prebiotic Foods as Prebiotic Foods

* Foods that are fermented.

* Avoid Antibiotics

* Avoid Antibacterial Cleaners

Make sure you eat a healthy diet with more than 60% fruit and vegetables.

The importance of Gut Health

There are approximately 22,000 human genes that reside in your body. However, most of Healthy Gut is very important. Microbiota, microflora, or Gut flora is present within our bodies at the moment we give birth and stays with us until we die. It aids in maintaining the normal and healthy state of our health.

Around the world Researchers are working on finding clues to the health and illness of humans. They have concluded that the cause of illness is Gut Health. The gut microbiota fights illnesses and helps maintain your mental and physical health. Gut health is vital to enhance the quality of your life in relation to ailments.

The microbiome, the beneficial bacteria in your gut. Gut bacteria is essential to maintaining well-being.

*The digestive system Gut is responsible for generating nutrients by breaking down foods we eat.

* Appetite -Gut microbes shape your appetite.

* Allergies fight against allergies.

* Metabolism: A higher metabolism is healthier.

* PsychologyIt has been discovered that gut bacteria affect your mood through the production of neurotransmitters such as serotonin, dopamine and GABA. The microbiota in your gut could fight off psychiatric diseases that are developing such as schizophrenia,

ADHD, obsessive-compulsive disorder, Somatoform Disorder, and chronic fatigue syndrome. The gut bacteria are crucial and influence how you feel.

Normal Health - The good bacteria within the Gut assist in maintaining the health of your body, which is extremely vital in our lives.

* Impact of the immune system A bad gut can impact the immune system, which leads to the body fighting itself. It is possible to develop food allergies due to the poor quality of the bacteria within the digestive tract.

* Inflammation- The bacterial found in the Gut could be the reason for inflammation. To reduce inflammation, you must have healthy bacteria in your Gut.

Conclusion:

Your gut microbiome is comprised up of trillions of bacterial, fungi , and other microbes. The gut microbiome plays an vital part in your health, aiding digestion control and improving your immune system, as well as other aspects of your health.

Things You Need to Be Educated About Gut Health

Our gut is home to millions of microorganisms to strengthen the immune system, and generating chemicals that make you feel happy and get energy from the food you eat. Today, Gut health has become an increasingly popular topic for doctors, scientists, and researchers. There are a lot of bacteria within our bodies, and it appears that the health of us is dependent on these microbes. The microbiome is the largest part of it is part of the biological process that determines our health and disease.

There is a loss of the diversity of their gut microbiome as a result of the change in our life style. Utilization of antibiotics, staying majority of the time inside, and unhealthy diet choices have led to the loss of diversity.

Each of us has a distinct "gut microbiome," which is like fingerprints that are produced in the house by around 160 species of bacterial.

When a baby enters the birth canal to give birth it is the initial location where microbes are brought to life. They are known as mother's microbes. They remain instabil bacteria as baby stage until they reach stability after two years.

As per the research they believe that the microbiome is an organ made up of microbes. However, at the exact it is true that microbiome plays a vital role in the Gut microbiome plays a vital function for our body's nervous system and immune system and the endocrine system. It is as much more than the above.

The gut microbiome is known as"your second brain. It is a Vagus nerve is connected to your brain , which alters your mood, happiness, and motivation, and can cause a suboptimal performance in your neurological abilities later on in your life. 90 percent of serotonin is created by microbes that act in the role of the "happiness brain transmitter." A healthy gut is connected with a healthy metabolism.

Antibiotics may alter the microbiota composition which can cause imbalance of microorganisms. This could have immediate and lasting effects on your health, particularly metabolism regulation as well as the immune system, and altering the microbiota's ecosystem over many years.

Important points to remember about gut health:

Relaxation is vital to maintain Gut health. There are a variety of methods to follow such as yoga or meditation to help you relax and the Gut and also.

"No news is always good news. If you're not experiencing any abdominal pains or sensations of the bloating sensation, then you're Gut is in good health and is healthy. Your Gut continually communicates with you about his well-being.

Whole foods should be consumed and we should avoid packaged or processed food items, which contain preservatives with no purpose that can disrupt the healthy bacteria living in the digestive tract.

*You should use fresh vegetables and fruits instead of canned fruits or vegetables.

However, frozen fruit can be healthy choices as long as no sugar or flavor is added.

*We should incorporate into our diet plenty of fiber, such as whole grains and legumes.

Probiotics are a good choice, like yogurt that is sugar-free.

For breakfast, we must cut down on the consumption of sugar. The addition of cinnamon to yogurt is added. It is worth considering Porridge and fresh Fruits, Oats with milk as different breakfast options.

*To maintain a healthful Gut it is recommended to include fermented foods like sauerkraut, kefir, or Kimchi.

*Eat a healthy balance of lean poultry and seafood as well as less red meat.

The Signs Of A Unhealthy Gut

The micro-biota that lives in our gut is essential to digesting food that we consume. It absorbs nutrients and then excretes the waste. Gutdysfunction happens because of an imbalance in the amount and diversity of the bacteria that reside within your Gut. Inadequate balance of the gut can affect the overall health of your body.

According to holistic health experts One of the main reasons why people aren't able to reap all the benefits of their superfoods-packed diet is due to invisible gut health issues that block the potent (and costly) substances from becoming consumed.

Every disease starts in the digestive tract. A lot of people who have digestive issues that make them feel tired, foggy and bloated. They also experience flatulence, constipation, nutritional deficiencies, diarrhoea weight gain, reflux, the inability to shed weight, cravings, lower immunity hormone imbalances. These symptoms can manifest as various chronic diseases , including obesity, diabetes, IBS, Chrohn's Disease and even depression and anxiety.

There are numerous blood tests, including ASCA, IBD profile and other tests like colonoscopy and endoscopy, to identify any anomalies in the function of the Gut.

Thus, ensuring digestive health and improving the gut's health is the main objective.

The Signs of a Poor Gut:

With our modern lifestyle, we have noticed increased stress levels, sleep deprivation and eating fast food as well as processed and high-sugar food as well as taking antibiotics. All of these have adversely affected and negatively impacted our Gut microbiome. The most evident indicators of a deteriorating Gut are listed below:

1. Stomach disturbances

The formation of gasand bloating diarrhoea and constipation. Pains in the abdomen, and heartburn are indicators of a sluggish stomach.

2. A high-sugar intake

Consumption of a high-sugar diet destroys a lot of beneficial bacteria that reside within your gut. The absence of good Gut bacteria makes your cravings increase and you'll start eating more food, which in turn damages your Gut flora. Consuming a diet high in sugar, specifically high fructose corn syrup can be the reason for inflammation of the body which can lead to fatal diseases such as cancer.

3. Weight imbalance

If you are losing weight with no mechanism for weight-management i.e. without a change in the diet or exercising routine, it could be due to an unhealthy digestive. Losing or gaining weight without making any changes to your exercise or diet routine could be an indication of a weakened gut. Unbalanced gut bacteria may hinder the capacity to absorb nutrients, control blood sugar levels as well as store excess fat. In excess, the growth of bacteria can be a cause of weight loss, and insulin resistance could be the cause of weight growth. In addition, insulin resistance can trigger the desire to eat more because of a lower absorption of nutrients.

4. Sleep deprivation

A man who is healthy must enjoy an uninterrupted sleep of eight hours. But, a poor stomach may be the reason that disturbs your sleep and cause you feel tired or suffer from poor sleep. Insomnia can lead to problems with depression, fatigue, and the capacity to live a an active and healthy lifestyle. The serotonin that is produced by the Gut can affect your the quality of sleep and mood. Gut flora that is not healthy can make it difficult to rest well.

5. Skin rashes, skin diseases and skin rashes

A damaged gut can affect the skin and may cause you suffer from skin disorders such as eczema. Inflammation of the gut resulted from inadequate diet or food allergy could lead to an increase in the leakage of specific proteins into the body. This could, in turn, create irritation on the skin and trigger skin conditions like eczema.

6. Autoimmune disorders

If autoimmune is overactive it causes inflammation in the intestine as well as other organs of the body , leading to various diseases such as Crohn's disease and irritable bowel syndrome, and irritable bowel. The bad bacteria that reside in the Gut can affect the immune system and affect the same process with inflammation and function of your immune system. This causes autoimmune conditions which cause your body to attack your body with no external stimulus.

7. Food intolerances

A low-quality bacteria that is that are not beneficial to our Gut causes food intolerance for certain foods, and, consequently it becomes difficult to digest certain kinds of food, creating symptoms like diarrhoea and gas abdominal pains, acid reflux and nausea.

8. You get sick often.

Your immune system is situated within your gut. Therefore, a weakened gut is a risk for illnesses frequently.

Conclusion:

The gut microbiome has become more crucial to be considered to ensure a healthy lifestyle. It's been a long time since the digestive system was thought of as a way to digest the food items and then eliminate the waste. Nowadays it is becoming more important to Gut is increasing every day to lead an active and healthy life free of preventable illnesses.

The bacteria in our homes are more than humans. Gut bacteria that are beneficial boost the immune system of your body, treat your depression, combat diabetes, obesity and many other benefits.

Chapter 2: What You Can Do That Can Harm Your Gut Bacteria

The negative side effects of our modern living is excessive stress, a lack of sleep, consumption of processed and high sugar food items. In addition, as we are taking the use of antibiotics all of these elements harm the microbiome of our gut. This can affect overall well-being and overall health.

With no healthy Gut microbiome, we've begun to suffer from various health problems, such as deadly diseases. It's affected our brain, heart and immune system, the skin, weight hormones, the ability to absorb nutrients or even the possibility of cancer.

There are many ways in which your microbiome could become unhealthy. Here are some of the ways your microbiome can be out of balance

1. Insufficiently having Diverse Foods

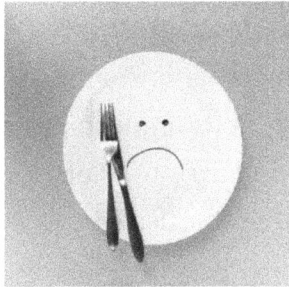

A diet lacking diverse whole foods can lead to an increase in the variety of Gut microbiota. It is essential to have a different kind of food, such as fruits, vegetables, as well as whole grains in order to have an increased diversity of gut microbiome. This will lead to an incredible experience. Yes! within 24 hours, your Gut flora begins changing its composition. The reason is that nutrients from food that help promote various kinds of bacteria that creates a diverse gut flora.

2.Using diet that does not contain Prebiotics

Prebiotics are a kind of fiber that circulates through the body without being digested and encourages the growth and activity of the friendly gut bacteria. A majority of vegetables, fruits, and whole grains are naturally rich in prebiotic fiber. It is important to include the following foods into our diet in order to reap the benefits of prebiotics.

Prebiotic-rich foods include:

* Lentils

* Chickpeas

* Beans

* Oats

* Bananas

* Jerusalem artichokes (looks like ginger)

* Asparagus

* Garlic

* Onions

* Nuts

3. Drinking Too Much Alcohol

If alcohol is consumed in massive quantities, it could be harmful to your wellbeing and health. If you prefer to drink, it is Red Wine.

Polyphenols in red wine assists to improve Gut health and helps to reduce harmful bacteria in the gut. It also reduces blood pressure and boosts cholesterol levels.

4. Use of Antibiotics

The use of antibiotics reduces the beneficial bacteria and prevents them from growing. It alters your microbe diversity that reside in the Gut. Although antibiotics can help in fighting infection excessive use can destroy the beneficial bacteria in your body. Probiotics will help to balance your body.

5. Physical inactivity

Physical exercise is a way to burn calories. The activity can change the gut microbiome, thereby improving health.

6. Cigarette Smoking

Smoke from tobacco is comprised of hundreds of chemicals, including 70 which could cause heart disease, cancer and more.

7. Not getting enough rest

A lack of sleep can affect your gut, brain and even your diet. Therefore, it is essential to take care to get enough rest. This is one of the major drawbacks of modern living.

Conclusion:

You're looking for and require good bacteria in your body. The good bacteria can aid in digestion as well as removing toxic substances from your body. They can keep your immune system healthy. So, stay clear of the factors mentioned above in order to ensure that your gut is healthy.

How to Restore Gut Health

Maintaining the gut health and maintaining the balance of microorganisms is crucial for mental and physical health, immune system and much more. Here are some ways to boost gut microbiome health and help improve digestion health.

1. Consuming probiotics and foods that are fermented and fermented

Research suggests that probiotics may help maintain the health of your gut microbiome, and that it can stop inflammation of the gut and other digestive issues. Fermented foods are an excellent food source for probiotics. In order to boost good bacteria known as probiotics in the digestive tract, some individuals choose to supplement their diet with probiotics. These can be found at pharmacies, health food stores, retailers, and even online.

2. Consuming Less Sugar

Consuming a large amount of artificial sweeteners and sugar can cause gut dysbiosis which refers to an imbalance of the microbes in your gut. Additionally research has revealed that artificial sweeteners can adversely affect blood glucose levels because of their impact on the gut flora. This is why they are to not be used at any times.

3. Eat fresh, unprocessed, whole foods.

Change to a whole food-based healthy, nutrient-dense diet. Remove food items that trigger inflammation, like dairy and gluten.

Additionally, a vegetarian diet can improve digestive health due to the prebiotic fiber that it has.

4. Treat any Intestinal Pathogens

Take care of any infections or an overgrowth of bugs. Small bowel bacteria, parasites and yeasts are all able to interfere with proper digestion. It is essential to treat these conditions for healing.

5. Get enough sleep

7 to 8 hours of quality sleep each night to maintain the health of your digestive system. Be sure to follow some good habits of good sleep, such as keeping a consistent sleep schedule and avoiding exposure to blue lights in the evening. Sleeping well can improve your mood, cognitive function and overall digestion.

6. A routine for exercise

Make a plan for a healthy exercise program to keep your gut microbes in good shape. Regular exercise is beneficial for health of the heart and weight loss or weight-maintenance. Studies have also indicated that it could boost gut health which could assist in the process of helping to reduce the weight gain.

7. Do not consume antibiotics unnecessarily

Antibiotics harm the gut microbiota as well as the immune system and immunity, with some studies revealing that after six months of their use, the gastrointestinal tract remains deficient of various beneficial bacteria. It is recommended to discuss alternatives to antibiotics with their physician prior to use.

8. Eat prebiotic fiber

Consume plenty of fermentable fibers that are found in various foods like onions, artichoke, garlic and plantains. These fibers aid in the development good gut bacteria and can help in healing leaky gut.

9. Manage Stress

Practice stress-reduction techniques like meditation or yoga, a element of your routine. Mindfulness apps like Headspace or Calm are beneficial for people who are just beginning to learn about meditation.

Conclusion: Improving digestion could take some amount of time but will be achieved. If you're looking to attain optimal health, focus on your digestion by following the above steps and observe how your symptoms diminish.

Disease Risk and Gut Health Connection

Hippocrates is reported as having said "death is a bowel issue" in addition to "bad digestion is at the root of all disease"

Many environmental influences could affect the intestinal microbial balance which has a strong relationship to health and illness. There is a constant interaction with the Gut microbiota as well as the body in a constant manner.

The microbiota's function is vital in the performance of fundamental biological functions and in the progression and development of human diseases of immense severity such as infectious diseases liver cancers, gastrointestinal cancers metabolic disorders respiratory diseases and mental or psychological disorders and autoimmune disorders.

The huge and active bacteria community is found within the Gut. The main roles of the microflora in our gut are metabolic functions that lead to the absorption of energy as well as the absorption of nutrients, and have important trophic impacts on intestinal epithelia as well as the function of immune cells and structure. They also protect against microbes that invade our gut.

All diseases originate within the gut. The bacteria in your gut and the gut lining can affect your well-being. Foreign molecules are detected by your immune system and are attacked which causes chronic inflammation. Inflammation is recognized as the root cause of numerous illnesses. Some of the conditions that are afflicted by bacteria that are unfriendly to the Gut are as follows:

Researchers have discovered links between bacteria and these illnesses:

* Irritable Bowel Syndrome

* Crohn's Disease

* Cancer

* Obesity

* Celiac Disease

* Colitis

* Diabetic

* Heard Disease

* Malnutrition

* Obesity

* Depression, and many other.

Chronic Inflammation

The immune system is able to respond to cell injury, toxins and foreign intruders it triggers inflammation. The immune system is designed to aid your body in fighting these unwanted invaders, and then repairing damaged structures.

But, in the short term, inflammation the duration of time, is healthy and also because you are able to recognize what actions to take as a response to an insect bite, bacteria or viruses that are affecting your health, or may even lead to death. However chronic inflammation can be harmful since it could impact the whole body.

Due to chronic inflammation, many illnesses can cause you to suffer from obesity, heart disease metabolic syndrome, diabetes depression, Alzheimer's disease Crohn's disease IBS, and many more.

Itchy Bowel Syndrome:

The interaction between the microbiota as well as genes leads to an ongoing inflammatory process that damages the mucosa in the intestinal. IBD is a condition that comprises Crohn's Disease (CD) along with ulcerative colitis (UC) has been suspected to result from an unnatural response to microbiome in the gut.

The Endotoxins as well as Leaky Gut

Two kinds of bacteria are found within our Gut. Certain of these bacteria are beneficial while others aren't. This means that the composition and number of your gut's bacteria can significantly affect your mental and physical well-being.

Liver disease:

Endotoxemia is a bacterium that causes negative effects which causes inflammation that can cause liver conditions, like the liver cirrhosis. The analysis of patients with cirrhosis showed lower levels of Bifidobacteria that are beneficial. The cirrhosis is linked to changes in gut microbiota.

Diabetes and Obesity

The overweight are more likely to be suffering from diabetes. The fluctuating levels of glucose can cause unhealthy cravings for sweeteners that increase our energy levels. In the end, due to the storage of excess glucose, an overflow of insulin blocks the signal to burn off the fat. Our beneficial bacteria boost the release of insulin in order to help us avoid diabetes-related issues.

Obesity is a multifaceted disease that results from interactions between genotype as well as the environment. The causes of obesity vary such as

* Environment

* Physiology,

* Metabolism

* Genetics

A poor gut can cause hormone imbalances that lead to diabetes and obesity.

Our hormones are supported by our healthy microbes. Leptin is the hormone that is responsible for the sensation of fullness. Leptin signals to the brain that it is full. This meaning that we shouldn't consume more. Thus, microbes increase the leptin's sensitivities, allowing our brain to have the sensation that we should not eat more. The excess of food can lead to obesity and diabetes.

Conclusion Gut flora is the primary factor in many illnesses that are pathological, such as multisystem organ insufficiency, colon cancer and inflammatory bowel disease. In addition, bacteria are beneficial to the health of humans. Probiotics and Prebiotics have a crucial role in the treatment and prevention of certain ailments.

The best probiotic foods for optimal gut health

The food and drinks you consume influences the health of your microbiome. The microbiome that lives inside your digestive tract is influenced by what you put into your mouth. Therefore, choosing the right foods is vital to maintain your Gut well-being.

Change your microbiota through changing eating habits. When you alter the food you consume, your body begins making new microbiota.

Furthermore, eating fresh vegetables and fruits makes the gut bacteria stronger and able to safeguard your health. Fruits, grains, and beans provide a favorable gut environment, while meat junk food, dairy products, junk food and eggs can be a cause of a negative gut environment.

Probiotics and Prebiotics Two gut-healthy compounds

The two terms -prebiotics and probioticsare getting more understood, so you've seen them.

Probiotics are beneficial gut bugs. Prebiotics are food for these bacteria.

Foods that have been fermented and supplemented fall in that category called Probiotics. The prebiotics source is present in vegetables, fruits along with whole wheat. The fiber is the most important component of prebiotics. Around 97 percent of Americans are having a sufficient amount of protein, however only 3percent of Americans consume the recommended 40 % of fiber daily. Fiber intake is crucial to Gut health. Our Gut microbes are able to extract the energy that fiber provides and nutrients, vitamins and SCFA that boost our immune systems, reduce inflammation, and help prevent overweight.

The role of Prebiotics and Probiotics in maintaining optimal Gut Health:

When you eat it, you're not just eating to improve your health, but to ensure good health for the microbiota in your gut. Prebiotics and probiotics are vital to bolster the gut flora and ensuring the Gut Health.

* Signs of bloating diarrhoea, bloating and other forms of inflammatory bowel diseases will improve if you follow the probiotic-rich diet.

If antibiotics are given the majority of our good bacteria are killed , along with the bad bacteria. Probiotics assist in replenishing the amount of beneficial bacteria.

* Probiotics improve the immune system by creating a barrier or assisting the growth of intestinal tissue stopping harmful bacteria from getting into the bloodstream. This ensures that the overall well-being of the immune system is protected.

* Probiotics are referred to in the context of Psychobiotics in the context of brain chemical mentioned. Diets that are rich in Probiotics assists in the production of neurotransmitters, like serotonin and GABA and GABA, which regulate mood. Therefore depression can be treated by improving the health of your gut through control of the microbiome through eating a diet that is rich in probiotics from nature.

* If the microbiome in your gut is balanced and well-nourished it may help improve many of the signs that are associated with autoimmune diseases.

* Prebiotics helps your good bacteria to develop. Oats, bananas, flaxseeds, Garlic come under the category of prebiotics that are beneficial to Gut Health and help in protecting us from various ailments.

Cleaning the system:

There are two kinds of fibers: soluble and insoluble.

Soluble fiber can help lower blood glucose levels as well as LDL cholesterol. It is found in legumes, oatmeal, as well as some vegetables and fruits. In contrast insoluble fiber is helpful to cleanse the digestive system that is found in whole grains as well as kidney beans. It is also present in fruits and vegetables.

In the case of gut disorders, they can be corrected by a Fiber diet and Prebiotics:

The fiber diet plays an important part to reduce inflammation in the intestinal tract. Insoluble fiber can help reduce the chance of developing disease due to inflammation in the intestine.

Fermented Foods: In addition to your diet the fermentation foods can also improve your gut health. Fermented foods eliminate bad gut bacteria, improve the absorption of minerals and boost well-being.

If we include the following fermented foods into our diet, they will help improve overall health, digestion, and immunity. gut health.

1. Sauerkraut

Sauerkraut is made of the cabbage and salt. This fermented food provides a healthy amount of probiotics as well as fiber.

2. Kefir

It is a drink made from fermented milk. It has the taste of a drinkable yogurt. Kefir is a great source of nutrients like calcium as well as probiotics. Similar to yogurt, the probiotics in kefir aid in breaking down lactose, which means it is more digestible for those with lactose intolerance. Kefir is great in smoothies or on its own.

3. Kimchi

This dish of fermented cabbage is spicy.

4. Kombucha

Kombucha is a sweet sparkling tea, typically green or black that is rich in beneficial yeast and bacterial. It is usually flavored by adding fruit or herbs. Kombucha can be found in natural food shops, farmers' markets and even your local supermarket. A small amount of alcohol may be created in the process of fermentation.

5. Miso

A fermented paste made of rice, barley or soy beans, miso imparts an umami-like flavor to food items. It's strong, and just a tiny amount can go far (which is beneficial since it's also very high in sodium). Miso is usually used in soups, however, it also makes the salad dressings, marinades and sauces more tasty and healthy for your gut.

6. Tempeh

Tempeh is made from soybeans that are naturally fermented. It's similar to tofu because is a protein derived from plants derived of soy, however, unlike tofu it's fermented. Also, the tempeh has a softer texture and a slightly sweeter taste. It's a great source of probiotics. And, since it's a complete source of amino acids, is a full vegetarian protein source.

7. Yogurt

The process of making yogurt is by fermenting milk. Yogurt that is branded with the "Live and Active Cultures" seal will guarantee 100 million probiotic bacteria per grams (about 17 billion in a 6 ounce cup) during the manufacturing process. Even the yogurts that do not have this seal have probiotics. Probiotics in yogurt can help to digest some lactose (milk sugar) which means that those who are lactose intolerant could be able enjoy yogurt. In addition numerous companies are offering vegan and dairy-free yogurt products that have probiotics.

Conclusion:

You can feed the probiotics in your gut by taking prebiotics, which are indigestible, digestible fibers that are the belly bugs' preferred food source. Consume honey, oatmeal and bananas, asparagus and onions. You can also add the daily dose of a prebiotic powder to provide the best support.

Chapter 3: The Spices To Enhance Your Digestion And Gut

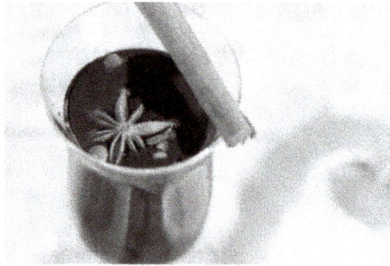

Role of spices in digestion:

Spices have been used in the ages to stimulate digestion.

Recent studies have revealed that a variety of foods stimulate the liver which results in the release of the bile which has a higher proportion of Bile acids. Bile acids are crucial in fat digestion and also absorption, therefore making sure that you've got enough is crucial.

Certain spices also assist in improving food transport time in the digestive tract. A slow GI tract can allow more liquid to absorb by the food digested, which may cause constipation that is painful. In addition, the longer the digested food items are allowed to be in your system prior to when it's eliminated more likely to be taken advantage of by harmful bacteria.

Some of the Top Spices to help digestion

1) Ginger

Ginger is a rich source of phenolic compounds that are believed to ease gastrointestinal irritations. It boosts the production of saliva and bile. Ginger eases intestinal contractions by relaxing abdominal muscles, allowing the digested food to pass through more easily. It also reduces the cramping of the stomach as well as the bowels, and can even assist menstrual cramps.

Ginger is effective in the reduction of gas and bloating. It is renowned for treating other stomach-related issues like nausea due to morning sickness or chemotherapy. Contrary to

Dramamine which is known to cause nausea, ginger can help reduce nausea but without making you feel sleepy.

2) Coriander Seeds/Cilantro

Coriander seeds, which produce cilantro are extensively used over the years to aid in digestion. Both coriander seeds as well as cilantro are healthy, however these seeds offer more benefits to digestion.

Coriander is carminative which means that it assists in gas production. It also is known for its stomachic and antispasmodic properties. It eases the spasms in the intestines that could lead to diarrhoea. Therefore, it could be beneficial to those suffering from an irritable bowel syndrome.

In addition It is also a source of phytochemicals, which are great antioxidants. Cilantro has also been studied for its potential as a detoxifier of heavy metals.

3.) Cardamom

Cardamom belongs to the family of ginger, and it's there's no reason to doubt that it can help digestion. It's been used for centuries in Chinese and Ayurvedic medical practices for centuries, but is also confirmed by science as having properties which help ease gas and bloating (aka carminative effects).

Cardamom can also increase appetite and helps ease nausea, gas and cramping. It assists in killing any food-borne bacteria that may be found in your digestive tract thereby protecting against gastric discomfort.

Cardamom pods contain a chemical known as limonene. It's commonly found in the citrus peels. It is known to dissolve cholesterol-containing gallstones, as well as relieve heartburn and gastroesophageal reflux (GERD).

4) Fennel Seeds

Fennel is a stimulant for in the creation of stomach juices. It is a great spice that has carminative properties. It is frequently utilized as a digestive aid. Also, it is antispasmodic. qualities.

Fennel seeds are an extremely high source of fiber in your diet and. It is composed of insoluble, metabolically inert fiber, which means it boosts the quantity of foods you consume when it passes through your digestive tract. It helps ease constipation. Fiber assists in protecting your colon.

Other important spices are:

Turmeric The Indian spice helps with digestion and relaxing the digestive system. It's been shown to ease stomach pain, relieve heartburn (due due to the anti-inflammatory and antibacterial properties) as well as reduce flatulence and many more.

Cumin -Cumin - Cumin is a excellent digestive spice that is excellent for heartburn.

Lemon Balm -- One of my most-loved digestive spices are lemon balm!

Garlic • Garlic helps to boost gut immunity.

Fenugreek -Fenugreek works as a natural digestive agent and assists in flushing out toxic substances from the body.

Cinnamon Bark - Warming the cinnamon bark is a moderate but beneficial treatment for constipation. According to the German Commission E recommends it to combat a lack in appetite, dyspeptic symptoms as well as bloating and flatulence.

Supplements to Gut Health

Function of Supplements

As we have discussed, to ensure that we keep our Gut well, we require probiotics that perform tasks that are beneficial to our health. Probiotics assist in eliminating harmful and unwelcome particles from our bodies. Thus, a gut-to-gut barrier is crucial to guard against harmful bacteria from our bodies.

These supplements are utilized to treat specific GI problems as well as for general health of the digestive system. Probiotics of various kinds can alleviate diarrhoea symptoms and also help relieve the symptoms of IBS or irritable bowel syndrome. (IBS).

These Probiotic supplements will help maintain the integrity of your Gut barrier and help promote the growth of beneficial bacteria that will help support your health today and in the future.

1. Enzymes

Enzymes are created by our bodies, and they aid in the breakdown of food. As we age our body's production of enzymes diminished. This decrease in enzymes result in less absorption of nutrients from our diet. The intake of plant-based supplements increases your digestion capacity and improves your overall energy levels.

Vegetables, fruits and fruit are the best source of enzymes.

2. Aloe Vera

Aloe Vera can be beneficial to the health of our gut. It falls under the category of prebiotics. It's a rich source of amino acids, as well as vitamins. It also assists in forming the gut barrier, and fights against constipationand inflammation. The supplement serves the function as a wiper of bad bacteria that reside in the Gut.

3. Acacia fiber

In addition, it is high in soluble fiber. Acacia fiber comes by the juice from the Acacia Senegal tree. It is a plant native to areas of Africa, Pakistan, and India. It is often referred to by the names of Gum Arabic and Acacia Gum, Acacia fiber is said to have numerous health advantages. Acacia fiber is a great prebiotic. This supplement aids in the reduction of weight , and helps reduce inflammation.

4.Fish Oil

It is believed that the Omega-3 of fish oils acts as an anti-inflammatory supplement that reduces intestinal inflammation. The fatty acids found in fish oil are also beneficial probiotics.

5.Butyrate

Butyrate salts can be made through distillation of vital oils that are extracted from vegetables. Gut bacteria also make this fat acid. It's beneficial for the colon cells since it provides nourishment and helps reduce inflammation within the digestive tract. Butyrate can also be found in butter made from grass and is sold as an added supplement.

6.Chamomile

This can be found through flowers. It is used as a medication in flower remedies therapy. It helps improve digestion, reduce gas and constipation. It also eases constipation.

7.Curcumin Phytosome

Curcumin, also known as turmeric is a yellow-colored herb commonly used to enhance taste and to maintain Gut health. It is also referred to as an anti-inflammatory herb that helps to reduce inflammation since the property of this plant are antioxidant. It functions as a barrier for the Gut.

8.Quercetin

Quercetin is an antioxidant flavonoid found in apples, onions along with citrus fruits. It functions as tight junction proteins, which perform the function of sealing the gap within the Gut barrier, thus safeguarding our body from microbes as well as other particles that might otherwise pass through.

9.Resistant Starch

Bananas, potatoes and legumes function as resistant starch. It is able to reach your colon intact to enrich the Gut filled with beneficial bacteria, which allows the beneficial bacteria to create short-chain fatty acids, such as butyrate. It also increases the sensitivity of insulin, which increases metabolism.

10. Slippery Elm

Slippery Elm is made from the elm tree in America. It's a mucilage-based substance that's used for protecting and soothing the digestive tract. It also functions as an antioxidant to relieve the symptoms of temporary inflammation. It can be helpful in cases of constipation and diarrhoea.

11.Vitamin D3

Vitamin D3 acts as an anti-inflammatory ingredient in the gut. It aids in improving the diversity of the microbiome in your gut and eliminates bad bacteria. Vitamin D3 aids in convert glucose into insulin for better sensitivity.

12.Zinc

Oysters and beef, as well as nuts and beans are all rich in Zinc. It's a class of minerals that provide significant protection walls for your stomach. A lack of Zinc can lead to damage to the intestinal membrane.

Gut feelings: Believing in your intuition

It is the mind that influences different glandular secretions. 80percent of all illnesses begin in the our minds. There is an automatic reaction of our body to a variety of stimulating agents. Eyes are shut quickly in response to eye-threatening stimuli. Also, when we experience an unusual or troubling situation the stomach becomes upset.

A good example of this is what we may have encountered when children experience loose movements during the exam days due to the anticipation of stress on the way they'll perform. The body reacts to any unwelcome event. The sensation of a tenseness is experienced when you hear negative news. The brain and gut affect one another. Brain-related emotions are felt by our Gut. Thus both the brain as well as Gut are inexplicably connected.

It is also a part of the brain:

It is believed that the job that Gut plays in Gut is to move food that we consume, digest, mixing juices and providing nutrition however, now scientists are discovering that Gut's functions Gut are so intricate that it contains over five times the number of as many neurons when compared with our spinal. The neurons that make up our nervous system, which is also known as"the brain with the 2nd. The second brain is situated within our Gut that sends signals to our brains which may relate to the immune system, appetite and many more.

Vagus Nerve connects the brain to the body.

It is the Vagus nerve serves as the one which connects the brain with the Gut. It sends messages to the brain, and the reverse. It lets the brain receive information. The majority of the fibers within the vagus nerve relay information through to the Gut and brain. Through this system of communication, Gut and brain stay connected. The amount of good or bad bacteria is contingent in the degree of the communication with Gut as well as Brain.

Your Brain's Microbiome:

The gut flora that you have is beneficial to your health and helps to make many neurotransmitters. These neurotransmitters aid your nervous system send messages to your brain, thereby providing a positive or negative sensation to your mood. Below are some salts that can improve your mood, based on the gut's signals.

* GABA.

Gaba is a salt that relaxes, made by Gut microbes. It helps ease nervousness, irritability and anxiety.

.* Cortisol.

Cortisol is an hormone that is elevated when you're stressed. Beneficial Gut flora reduces cortisol.

* Serotonin.

Gut bacteria create around 95% of serotonin , which is widely known for its positive chemical. It influences our mood and appetite, sleep, and memory.

* Dopamine.

The positive feeling you feel when you take substances, food as well as sexual stimulants is caused via the release of a variety of neurotransmitters in your brain, such as dopamine.

* Oxytocin.

A healthy level of the hormone oxytocin, which is aided by Probiotics boost feelings of affection and bonds.

What Does Your Gut Say to You?

Prior to thinking about it, you're is preparing your body to ensure that you're ready to react immediately. In this scenario, feeling the feeling of butterflies in your stomach after the first sound of the phone may signal that blood is being pumped out of the digestive system to your extremities, which allows you to act immediately. When you're under stress and you begin to feel unease and discomfort within your Gut convey the message that he's not content with the anxiety.

How to trust Your Gut Feelings

Gut health is a source of nutrition and helps guide you. It creates chemicals that alter your mood, and also communicate through your brain. Intuition, also known as gut instinct is your instant understanding of something. There's no need to consider it or ask for a second opinion. You simply already know.

The intuition you have is the sensation in your body that you are the only one to experience. Since the experience is individual, nobody other person can determine if you're connected to your instincts or not. Only you are the one who can make the decision. This is why faith in your instincts is the best way of being a good friend to yourself.

52

Take a moment to slow down and clear Your Mind. It is rooted in the bodily sensations that are inside the body, therefore it is important to sense what's happening inside your body--i.e. the sensations you're experiencing. Your intuition can be similar to an ocean current that guides you towards a meaningful life. Keep in mind that trusting your instincts is a process that can lead you back to these steps frequently as your the circumstances change and your life continues to evolve.

The Gut-Brain Axis

The gut-brain-axis refers to the chemical and physical connections between your brain and gut. Millions of neurons and nerves are connected between your gut and the brain. Neurotransmitters and other chemical substances produced within your gut can also impact the brain. If you can alter the types of bacteria that reside in your gut it could be possible to improve the health of your brain.

Omega-3 acid, fermented food Probiotics, as well as other foods rich in polyphenols can improve the health of your gut which can benefit in the gut-brain connection.

Chapter 4: The Inside Story How The Know Your Gut

What is the most recent time you've heard "trust your intuition"? You could also think of this "gut sensation" to be our sixth sense, or intuition. It is that intense, unfathomable feeling that is a part of the body. It can manifest itself as that butterflies-in-your-stomach excitement, or that sick-to-your-stomach kind of fear. Did you know there is a scientific reason behind these "gut feeling"? Scientists have found that the digestive (GI) tract also known as the gut, is home to an "second brain" also known as"the enteric nervous system (ENS). The system is composed of millions of nerve cells and which are part of the ENS connects with your brain inside your head, a process known by the term "brain-gut link" (or "gut connection between brain and gut."

Although we typically consider the gut to be the body organ responsible for breaking into food particles, the gut is actually responsible for many other duties. There are many ways in which the GI tract can influence different systems in the body. Knowing how gut health affects general health can give you an understanding of the reason why maintaining the health of your gut is vital.

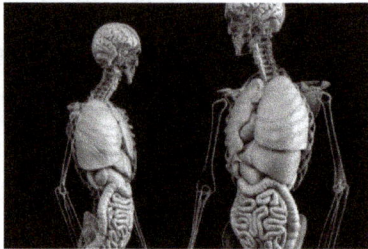

How do you define the Gut?

"The gut" is a broad word which refers to the digestive tract (GIT). The gastrointestinal tract extends from the mouth all the way into the anus. It is also called the digestive tract, or alimentary canal, it is component of digestion. The GIT is comprised of a muscular hollow tube that is located in the mouth where food is absorbed via the mouth. This tube is comprised of various muscles and components that assist in coordinating the movement of food throughout the body. After swallowing, food moves through the tube and is subjected to different processes before being eliminated.

When food passes across into the GI tract, various hormones and enzymes release throughout your body to help prepare digestion of the nutrients. Other cells like absorptive cells as well as Paneth cells (located within the intestinal tract) can be activated in order to aid in the breakdown of foods and the absorbance of nutrition. As you'll discover the GIT plays an important role in the various processes of the body. Its roles range from controlling sleep and stabilizing mood , to maintaining blood sugar levels and blood pressure in the right place.

The GI tract measures around 9 meters long, and it is folded to fit perfectly in the body. If the organ were to be folded, it would be the length of the length of a tennis court. The GIT comprises approximately 70% of our immune system, and is home to more than 4 tons of bacteria. The bacteria that live there are a key element in determining the effectiveness and health of the GIT. The dimensions of the gastrointestinal tract can give you an idea about how vital it is for the health of your body.

What is the Gut's Job?

The principal function of the digestive tract can be to digest food and release vital nutrients that are taken in through the body. The water and nutrients that are absorbed from our diets give the body with energy and keep it in good health. There are three main roles that the gut was created for, and our gut health directly influences how well it can perform these.

Principal Objectives

There are three main roles of the stomach which influence the way that other organs of the body function. The primary functions of the gut are digestion, transport as well as absorption and digestion of foods.

Food transportation: First, food items must pass through the mouth cavity, in order to be taken care of by the teeth, and then is softened by saliva. Food is swallowed , then moved down the esophagus until it is absorbed by the stomach, where it is stored temporarily. A one-quarter of a quart of food items can be saved in your stomach. It produces acid to help to break down food. There aren't many nutrients that are taken in by the stomach. Instead it is absorbed when the muscles start to contract and push it into the small intestinal.

Digestion: The process of digestion is primarily carried out in the small intestine , but starts within the stomach. In the stomach , food is combined with acid to initiate the process of breaking food down so it can easily be divided into nutrients.

Carbohydrates begin the process of digestion within oropharynx. The enzyme, serum amylase found in saliva, starts to break sugar molecules. The glucose and water are taken from carbohydrates through a process of going through the mucosa.

Absorption: The majority of nutrients are absorbed by the small intestine, where nutrition is broken down to most fundamental building blocks. The molecules are then passed through the epithelium or the wall in the small intestines, and get into the bloodstream. The large intestines are also involved in the absorption of excess water.

Aspects of the GI System

The gastrointestinal tract is made up of various components that travel through the body. The passageway is commonly known as the alimentary canal. It is a simple way to trace the path that our food items take. The entrance to this canal is called the mouth. Continue reading to find out where the food you consume is going to go.

The mouth is the part that comprises the oral cavity that is where digestion starts. Mouths are lined by the oral mucosa squamous and covering of keratin to guard against the areas that are more delicate and susceptible to scratching.

Food particles are broken down via the process known as mastication, which is the actual eating and chopping performed by teeth. It is the tongue's muscle which helps to manipulate food so that it can come into contact with teeth. The tongue also has a number of sensors that enable us to determine temperatures of food as well as feel different textures and distinguish the flavor of our food.

Pharynx: This is more commonly referred to for its throat. The pharynx actually performs the act of swallowing from the reflex. When food is swallowed, it will go through the pharynx before being transported into the esophagus. A portion of the pharynx connects towards the trachea, or windpipe, which absorbs air and then transfers it into the lung. After food is consumed in the pharynx the trachea is shut off to prevent food from passing through the wrong pipe.

Esophagus: It runs from the pharynx and into the stomach. It is a tube of muscle that measures about 10 inches in length and almost 1 inch in diameter. The tube's wall comprises of inner circular as well as the outer layers of muscle. There is a nerve-plexus that covers the lower portion of the esophagus. The main function of the esophagus's function is to move food from the mouth into the stomach.

Stomach The stomach is situated between the esophagus as well as the small intestine. It's a 'J" form that can expand to store more food. There are four major regions within the stomach. It is known as the cardia. This area constitutes the initial section that surrounds the entryway of the esophagus and the stomach. It is also the third section that connects with the diaphragm's left side. The third and biggest part in the stomach referred to as the "body. It lies in between the fundus as well as the round part that forms the J shape. Most gastric glands can be found within the stomach's body. It is also the place where the majority food mixing food items takes place. The last part is the pylorus, which is the curving base of the stomach.

The stomach is responsible for a range of functions, which include:

* temporarily storing food items

Mixing food in order to start break it into pieces

* digesting proteins with acids and enzymes

* creating acid that kills off the majority of bugs and germs ingestion

* absorption alcohol

Small Intestine: Small intestinal tract can be as long as the length of six metres. In the small intestines nutrients start to be absorbed into the bloodstream. The food mix that is passed by stomach travels through three different parts in the small intestinal tract. The three components are the duodenum, jejunum along with the ileum. Each of them plays a part in mixing the digestive fluids with the food and in breaking it down to aid in digestion. The duodenum is in which bile released from the intestine's walls mix with the fluids released by the pancreas. The mixture is then passed through the jejunum, where meals are reduced into vital nutrients (carbohydrates fat, carbohydrates, protein, and fat). The food then travels into the ileum where the majority of the water and nutrients are absorbed into the bloodstream. Anything that isn't absorption-related will move through the large intestine.

Large Intestine intestinal tract curves around the small intestinal tract and measures about 1 1/2 meters long. Large intestines are responsible for the transformation of non-absorbed matter into Feces. The large intestine is home to bacteria that release gas and reabsorb water sugar, salt and vitamins.

The rectum forms a component of the large intestine located in the final five inches. The primary function of the rectum is to keep the fecal matter until in good condition to pass by the anus. Muscles that create a band around the rectum regulate the flow of waste.

Other Organs

Other organs can also assist in digestion. The liver is filtering system for blood that is pumped through the digestive tract. This organ is responsible for detoxifying of metabolites as well as making albumin. Additionally, the liver plays an important part in the production of bile as well as processing nutrients. The nutrients that are absorbed by the intestines pass through the liver before being processed and then transported to the the body. The gall bladder is responsible for storage of bile produced by liver.

The pancreas plays a crucial role in making hormones like insulin. Cells in the body depend on insulin for the absorption of nutrients from food particularly carbohydrates. The pancreas is also accountable for the production of specific enzymes to help breakdown various food components that are going through the digestion process.

The Brain-Gut Connection

You might have heard about the "second brain that refers towards the stomach. The gut and brain share unique bidirectional connections which allows signals coming from the brain and the gut to be sent directly from each other. The communication between the gut and brain is carried out via the brain gut axis. The findings of new research have shown the brain-gut axis be a much more intricate communication system than we had previously believed.

In the past the brain-gut relationship was confined to the understanding that the gut and the brain sent signals that were related to the intake of food and digestion. For instance, we understand the fundamentals of this connection. The brain transmits signals for the GIT to initiate digestion. If the stomach is full the signalling is sent out to the brain to end food intake. The most popular route of signals transmitted between the gut and the brain was thought by the sympathetic nerve systems. This system controls our fight or flight response. Signals could also be transmitted through the parasympathetic nervous system that are responsible for our digestion and resting responses.

We now know that the communication between gut and brain is more intricate. Signals are transmitted through multiple systems within the body. Certain signals are transmitted through the nerve system while others are sent through the autonomic nervous system, and more through an enteric nerve system. The hypothalamic-pituitary-adrenal axis also comes into play. Knowing this connection can be essential and could help you understand what is causing you to struggle with health issues that, from a distance may appear to be unrelated to the digestive tract.

Internal Communication Between Gut and Brain

The brain-gut connection and the gut grows further than processing food, and controlling the appetite. The signals that are sent to and from these two areas affect the gastrointestinal homeostasis. The state of homeostasis is one where all functions and interactions within the gastrointestinal tract work correctly and in sync. The brain-gut is also a contributing factor to greater or lower cognitive functioning. The brain-gut-axis connects our emotional and cognitive function to digestive functions.

To know how signals are sent in both directions, we have examine the mechanisms these signals travel through. As we mentioned, communication is possible through Central nervous system the autonomic nervous system, the eccentric nervous system, and hypothalamic pituitary adrenal system. There are a variety of biological and physical connections between the gut and the brain.

The vagus nerve for instance is the longest-running nerve in the human body. It connects in the gut to the brain. It physically connecting the two and permits signals to travel to both sides. The gut is a biochemical source of several neurotransmitters. The most prominent of these is gamma-aminobutyric acids (GABA). GABA helps to control emotions, such as anxiety and fear.

The signals sent between the gut and the brain influence the way food passes through the digestive tract. This also affects the intake of nutrients, the production of digestive juices and levels of inflammation within your digestive tract. A healthy gut can result in improved physical and mental well-being. An increasing amount of research is underway to gain a better understanding of these conditions as well as how the gut-brain connection could shed new light on the treatment of certain neurological disorders.

A recent area of study focused on the brain-gut relationship is on our gut's microbiota. The gut is comprised in millions of microorganisms that are present throughout all of the intestinal tract. The group of microorganisms comprise the microbiota of the gut. They help to regulate the immune system's response and produce hormones and affect the overall health of our body. Researchers are investigating the role of the digestive tract in playing an important role in the development of certain diseases and how improving the health of our gut can aid in preventing, battling or reverse some ailments that stem from the bacteria that reside within your digestive tract. In the next chapter we will go over the most recent findings regarding how these microbes impact the health of our digestive tract and overall health.

You now have a good knowledge of what your gut is, the functions it performs, and the much it influences general health. You will also discover that there are many different types of guts that are not identical. Although the functions and parts that comprise the stomach are similar for every person but the process of digestion differs little between women and men. It is also evident that there are distinct variations in the functions of the intestines as we get older.

How well do you know Your Gut?

Try this short test to test your knowledge of the concepts you've discovered in this section. Take the test without looking back or looking at the answers that is below.

1. The digestive tract starts in the _____.

A. the throat

B. the stomach

C. the mouth

2. The stomach is made up of what number of parts?

a. 5

b. 1

c. 2

d. 4

3. The three major components are duodenum, jejunum and _____.

A. diaphragm

b. ileum

C. Pylorus

4. The pathway of communication between the gut and the brain is known as?

a. brain-gut axis

B. sympathetic nervous system

c. esophagus

5. What are microorganisms which are found in the digestive tract?

A. Large intestine

B. the bloodstream

C. microbiota

(Answers: 1. c. 2. d. 3. b. 4. a. 5. c)

Chapter 5: Find The Different How Gender And Age Affect Your Gut

Although our digestive system of females and males are similar in many ways, they have crucial differences that can influence the way in which they react to how they react to medication and food. One of these differences was revealed in a study which revealed women are slower to digest food than men. It took on average 33 hours for males to digest food, and an average of 47 minutes for women (Women and men differ in terms of digestion in 2020). The slower flow of food through our system results in women experiencing more digestive problems in general as compared to males.

Alongside the gender difference in addition, the digestive tract (GI) alters with the advancing years. Understanding the differences between GI tracts is crucial to know the best ways to take treatment of your gut today and over the next few years. It's also crucial since as we age, other issues arise which can affect digestion. Women who are going through menopausal changes will be experiencing diverse digestive problems due to hormonal changes. It's also becoming more crucial to take care of your digestion to prevent osteoporosis and other age-related diseases that are more likely to occur for women who are older than 50. Being aware of what is to expect as you get older will help you adopt preventive measures to prevent serious health problems from occurring before they are required.

Male Vs. Female Gut

Females and males differ in physiology and physiology in various ways. This includes the way your digestive tracts constructed and positioned as well as how they function. Although the procedure itself is identical but there are some significant distinctions that cause digestion to be more complicated for women. There are also a variety of differences in the digestive system that place women at greater risk of specific digestive problems and place men at higher chance of developing other.

We'll begin near the start of our digestive tract in the esophagus. The esophagus is exactly the same for women and men. The major distinction between them has something to do with the entrance that is located between the esophagus as well as the stomach. For women, this opening is closed with greater force than in men and ensures that when food is passed through the esophagus, and then into the stomach, it's quickly held in place.

There are a few variations when we reach the stomach area of stomach and digestive tract. women produce less stomach acid than men, and that is the reason they are less prone to damage to the stomach. However, stomach inflammation , or gastritis is more frequent for women. The reason for this is that food stays within the stomach longer than males. As the stomach starts to empty, food takes longer to drain out from the stomach. Women experience more nausea and bloating as a result of the slower digestion process of food.

The colon also drains slower in females. The female colon is about 4 inches larger that the colon of a male. The difference in size leads to slow release of contents of the colon.

Womenare, therefore, more likely to experience IBS, also known as irritable bowel syndrome (IBS)--also known as chronic constipation. IBD, also known as inflammatory intestinal disease (IBD)--also called the rapid movement of bowel.

Another major distinction is the location of the colon inside the body. Male colons are situated over the abdomen while it is in the same place as the reproductive system. The colon is interwoven with the uterus and the other reproductive organs resulting in material passing through the colon to follow an increasingly winding and curled route. Women might have more issues in bowel movement after they are pregnant due to how the colon is situated within other reproductive organs.

Other Things to be aware Of

Here are some additional variations between women and men which can cause problems with digestion:

* Female hormonal fluctuation affects digestion. The changes in female hormones can lead to constipation, fluid retention constipation, constipation and slow digestion. It can take as long as 14 hours more time for food to travel through the female's large intestine as compared to a male.

• Men tend to be suffering from heartburn and acid reflux because their stomachs are awash with acid. If acid is released from the stomach often, it could cause harm to the esophagus.

* Women are at greater chance of developing dyspepsia (pain on the upper abdomen) that can lead to nausea and bloating.

* Women are more likely to use prescription anti-inflammatory medications that can cause stomach irritation and result in ulcers.

The likelihood of women being more susceptible to experience IBS or irritable IBS (IBS). IBS is a cause of several digestive issues like bloating and gas, excess gas along with constipation, diarrhea, and constipation. The male hormones produced by men can provide them with extra protection from the condition. However women don't produce as or more many as these hormonal substances. In addition, estrogen and progesterone the female hormones can contribute to the worsening of signs of IBS. If the concentrations of the hormones are elevated, women can experience more abdominal bloating and constipation.

The Age Factor

Many organs and systems of our bodies start to undergo rapid changes and decrease in their proper functioning. The positive side is that the gut is more likely to be spared the effects of aging when as compared to organ systems throughout the body. But, the gut will be affected by aging. These changes typically appear as a diminution or slowing of the functions as well as an increase in the chance of developing digestive tract problems. According to a study more than 40% of seniors suffer from age-related changes to their digestive tract once they reach the threshold of age 65 (Comaway 2012).

Alterations to GI Changes to the GI We Age

While you may not be able completely prevent the effects of aging but you will be aware of what to look for. Because the digestive tract is composed of a variety of individual parts, it is possible to suffer from multiple age-related ailments for each one as well as conditions that affect the digestive system in general. Knowing the effects of age on the digestive tract can put you in a position to take a proactive approach to keeping your gut in good shape well into your 70s or 60s. The changes in certain parts that comprise the GI systems can become more obvious as we get older. They could include:

• Mouth. We are likely to have more trouble swallowing and chewing as we get older due to our jaw muscles becoming weaker. Also, we produce less saliva, which makes it difficult to swallow certain foods , and demands more energy from the the digestive system to break down foods.

* Esophagus: muscles which manage those contractions as well as tension within the esophagus begin to weaken. It is not uncommon for this to affect the ability of the

esophagus to transport food. However, it could occur due to other conditions that can affect the function of the esophagus.

* Stomach: There are couple of changes that happen to the stomach with get older that could affect our digestion. First, the lining the stomach loses its elasticity with time. This makes it difficult for our stomachs to absorb the amount of food it did in the past. The stomach is also more susceptible to damage and ulcers are more likely to develop which can cause discomfort and pain.

* Small Intestine Lactase an enzyme created in order to breakdown lactose decreases with time. This could result in lower tolerance to dairy products. Low lactase levels can also affect the growth of bacterial cells, which can affect how our bodies absorb specific nutrients. It is not unusual for women over 50 to suffer deficiencies in calcium, iron and vitamin B12.

"Large Intestine": When you get old, it requires longer time for food to pass across the large intestinal tract. The slower passage of foods through our large intestine leads to an increase in the amount of water that is absorbent. This could cause constipation to become more frequent.

* Rectum: It grows bigger as we age, and muscle contraction diminishes. The result is a rise in episodes of constipation.

Age-related issues of the GI Tract

Gastrointestinal problems and digestive issues are more commonplace when we reach the age of 65. These issues may be moderate to mild and some are more severe. It is crucial that if you have any of the conditions listed below, you speak to your doctor and start taking effective actions to decrease the likelihood of developing further issues.

* Heartburn: The heartburn may be a problem at any age , but it is more prevalent in older people. Heartburn is a feeling of burning in your chest. The cause of this pain is stomach acid moving through the esophagus, and then towards the mouth and throat. It is possible to notice the taste of sourness within your mouth. It can also make you or feel full, and your voice

could be strained. Heartburn can occur immediately after we eat and may last for several hours. When we lie down, the symptoms tend to get worse. As we age, muscles that line the lower part of the esophagus start to shrink, which makes the stomach acids easier to flow back into the tube, instead of remaining in the stomach region.

*Peptic Ulcers Peptic ulcers develop on the inside of the stomach lining, as well as in the openings in the small intestine. They can trigger extreme stomach discomfort.

* Gastrointestinal ulceration: Because older people tend to be more likely to use an array of medicines including anti-inflammatory drugs as well as heart medications and there is an increased chance of stomach bleeding.

* Diarrhea: Diarrhea is having the sudden and intense desire to go. If we do, the bowels are very unsteady. If our digestive tract isn't taking in nutrients in a proper manner, we may be suffering from diarrhea. Numerous lifestyle changes that happen as we age may also trigger more diarrhea . This could be due to not

drinking enough water, and decreasing physical activities. And disruptions to sleep patterns.

* Constipation: a third of older adults experience changes in their bowel movements. Constipation is among the most frequent digestive issues that people over the age of 60 face more frequently. There are many reasons why constipation can become more prevalent as you stages of. The first is that the digestive system processes food at a slower rate. It takes some period of time for food to be moved from one area of the tract and into the next. Once food gets to the colon it slows the process more , which causes more water to be absorption from the waste that we must get rid of. This causes dry or hard stool that is difficult to eliminate at the point of no return.

The slower digestion of food may also result in frequent constipation. It is possible that you experience pain as a result of constipation. Also, the medications you could take to treat other ailments can cause constipation as an adverse result.

Seniors who are taking medication to lower blood pressure are susceptible to suffering from constipation. Diuretics are usually used to reduce blood pressure and can result in an increase in the amount of urine that results in loss of fluids in the body. A lot of people not drink more fluids in order in order to reduce the frequency they require the bathroom. This means you have to eliminate more fluid and not replenishing what you've lost increases the chance of becoming dehydrated. If we're dehydrated, there won't be enough fluids in our digestive tract to allow waste to pass easily or comfortably, and cause constipation.

We also make less stomach acids as we get older and this means that our food is not being broken down properly before being transferred to the intestinal tract. This can slow digestibility and can make it harder to transfer food into the remainder of the tract.

* Hemorrhoids: Hemorrhoids occur when veins of the lower rectum get constricted or swollen. They may be found both externally and internally. Internal hemorrhoids might not

cause discomfort but tend to trigger bleeding. External hemorrhoids may be painful and can cause discomfort when standing or walking. Hemorrhoids are more prevalent as we age due to the support tissues in the rectum weakens and expands. If you experience constipation frequently, which is more prevalent as you get older, you're more likely to develop hemorrhoids.

"Gas:" The slowing of digestion may result in more gas being expelled from food items which are stored in the stomach, or other parts in your digestive tract. A slower metabolism could result in you becoming increasingly gassy and uncomfortable as you grow older.

• Stomach pain: Stomach discomforts can get frequently as you grow older. A slower digestion can weaken muscles along the digestive tract, as well as other medical conditions may contribute to greater abdominal discomfort.

*Irritable Bowel Syndrome (IBS): Women are more likely to develop IBS when they reach 50. IBS can cause stomach pains as well as irregular stool movements. There are many factors that are responsible for IBS which are not directly linked to the age. Exercise, diet, sleep and stress can increase the likelihood of developing IBS.

* Diverticulitis: When you reach 65 years old, you are at 50% higher chance to develop diverticulitis (Weizman and Nguyen 2011,). Diverticulitis is a condition in which tiny sacs expand out of the colon's outer wall into the weaker parts within the wall of your intestinal. It is common for them to appear in the lower region of the colon.

• Fecal Incontinence: It's not unusual for older people to experience difficulty controlling the flow of their bowels. The contraction and weakening of the muscles in the digestive tract could cause difficulty in keeping things in position. Incontinence feces are a frequent phenomenon in women during their menopausal phase. The low levels of estrogen or treatment for hormones can make it more likely that you will develop the condition known as fecal incontinence. Stress and anxiety may lead to having a temporary incontinence fecal.

* Gastroesophageal Reflux Disease (GERD) Reflux is a very common illness of the upper digestive tract. GERD is caused when stomach acid is rerouted back to the esophagus, which can trigger heartburn as well as other complications in stomach and upper gastrointestinal tract, such as chronic coughing and sore throat. Numerous lifestyle factors can trigger symptoms of GERD and a lot of them are not related to be related to age. Foods that are consumed late in the evening, fast food, or eating fried or fast foods frequently increase the likelihood of the frequency of reflux. Other factors related to age, like taking certain medicines can also increase the risk of reflux.

* Polyps: Polyps are tiny growths that occur within the colon. When you reach 50, you are at more of a chance of developing these tumors. Although many of them may be benign, some may develop into cancerous. A majority of the growth is not detected because it doesn't display any signs. This is why it's important to

undergo regular screenings, such as colonoscopies. It is crucial to identify these tumors and get them removed before they develop into cancerous.

* Colon Cancer: Colon cancer is a frequent problem for older people. The age at which for men who are diagnosed with the disease is 68. For women, it's around 72 (CancerNet Editorial Board 2021). Even with this higher mortality rate for women, it's crucial to schedule regular screenings to aid in detecting colon cancer beginning stages.

Be aware that the digestive tract is likely to show normal wear and tear as you get older. However, other health issues which are not directly connected to the digestive tract can accelerate the damage. Being proactive to maintain good health will ensure that your gut stays in good condition , regardless of stage of life.

We've now explained how gender and age influence the gut, it's time to start learning about gut issues that could lead to unhealthiness. The next chapter will start by exploring the factors that is affecting the health of your gut and discover why gut health that is healthy is crucial.

How Do You Know Your Gut?

After you have learned about the various digestive related issues you might be suffering from, take a look at the issues you could be experiencing. Consider a minute to write down any health concerns or ailments you are currently experiencing. They may be related to the bowels, stomach or even digestive discomfort. Don't ignore or dismiss issues since they're what you've always experienced. For instance, you might be used to feeling bloated when eating, and it's become a normal thing for you. However, it is still digestive discomfort. It doesn't make a difference how long, or short the time that you've felt the symptoms: take note of each and every one. This will be helpful in the coming chapters.

Additionally, list any other concerns or issues you might be experiencing that, for the moment may not have any connection with your digestion health. Take note of this list, you'll be amazed by what number of issues you write down are connected to your gut when you go through the rest of the book.

Be aware of your gut: Understanding the 'What' as well as the "Why" of an unhealthy GI

Two millennia ago Hippocrates the founder of modern medicine stated, "All disease begins in the gut." Nowadays the statement has been proven valid through numerous studies and deep research. While not all ailments originates from the digestive tract (GI) however, the GI can be a major contributor to or trigger many chronic illnesses.

A lot of people consider and just think that they'll be dealing with a myriad of digestive problems due to the food they consume. However, these issues could frequently be a sign for more serious health problems. Food is the main source of digestion-related issues however there are other factors that influence the stomach. Knowing what the triggers are can help you develop an effective plan for making essential changes that will improve your overall health.

89

A sign of a shaky gut

Numerous factors can impact digestive health. Things like sleep patterns food, diet, or stress can cause disruption to the digestion process. While certain issues with the gastrointestinal tract are evident, there are many ways in which an unhealthy gut may display symptoms. The most frequent symptoms of a shaky digestive tract are listed below.

Stomach discomfort: Issues such as excessive gas, constipation, bloating as well as diarrhea and abdomen pain are signs of an imbalanced stomach. The reason for these symptoms is that it is because the GI tract is struggling to digest food items properly and remove waste properly. This could be a sign of IBS. Unbalanced gut bacteria is typically the main source of many forms of stomach pain.

Cravings for food are usually a signal for your body to inform that it's lacking certain nutrients. However, these cravings can appear as an urge to eat foods that could cause harm to the digestive tract. The craving for sugar is an indication of an imbalance in the gut bacteria.

The harmful bacteria are able to feed on sugar. If there are more harmful bacteria in your gut, you'll feel more compelled to eat sugar since the bacteria need sugar to take advantage of.

* Tiredness or sleep disturbances If you are struggling to get to sleep or stay asleep, this could be due to an unbalanced gut. When we do not succeed in sleeping well, it is more probable that we experience chronic fatigue. Serotonin is the chemical responsible for sleep and relaxation is made by the gut. Melatonin is a particular type which is which is the natural aid to sleep is also made in the gut. If the gut isn't functioning properly , these hormones could not release at the right timing or the body might not be able to produce enough quantities to ensure a good night's sleep. Infection or dysfunction in the GI tract may interfere with this hormone production, which hinder sleep.

* Skin problems or irritations Skin conditions and irritations may indicate a poor digestive tract. Eczema is among the most prevalent skin disorders that develops due to damage to the digestive tract. The inflammation caused by

poor eating habits or food allergy are primary causes of the gut to be damaged. Damage is caused by the digestive tract failing to absorb certain proteins found in the food we eat. These proteins could escape from the GI tract and into the bloodstream, causing irritation to the skin and can cause other skin conditions such as eczema or the psoriasis.

* Autoimmune disorders In the event that the gut is not healthy, the immune system suffers. While further research is needed to better understand the relationship to the digestive tract and the immune system It is thought that inflammation in the digestive tract causes that the body's immune system fail to function properly. This can increase the chance of developing an autoimmune disease where the body start to attack the cells of its own in opposition to harmful invaders, such as viruses or bacteria.

Intolérances to food: These are due to the fact that the digestive system isn't able to process certain food items. Food intolerances result from inadequate gut bacteria, which hinders digestion's capacity take in certain foods. Constipation, abdominal pain nausea, diarrhea and gas are among the most frequent symptoms of food intolerance.

* Allergies food allergies differ from food intolerances as they are caused by the immune system that experiences a negative reaction to certain food items. As we've discussed the gut and the immune system are in close contact and food allergies could be influenced by the health of your gut.

Unpredictable mood swings The brain-gut link means that when the digestion is operating at a loss to function as it is supposed to, the brain could miss certain messages coming by various parts of the body. A lack of gut-friendly bacteria, an increase in inflammation, as well as a lack of absorption of nutrients could trigger disorders like anxiety and depression.

* Migraines: Migraines can be caused by an unhealthy gut. Women have three times the chance suffer from migraines frequently than males (Devlin 2016). Research has revealed that those suffering from migraines have an entirely

different set of gut bacteria and it's not a healthy combination. There is a higher percentage of bacteria that digest nitrates (often present in processed wine, meats and some vegetables with leafy leaves) could be the root cause for migraines. The bacteria could break down nitrate food items more effectively, and when the nitrate-rich food is processed, they are converted into the nitric oxide before it enters the bloodstream. Nitric oxide is believed for its ability to dilate blood vessels.. Because the blood flowing through the gut can swiftly travel to the brain through the brain-gut connection, the vessels of the scalp and the brain expand and cause migraines.

* Weight changes unaccounted for changes in weight could be an indication of a weakened gut. Weight loss or gain which isn't caused by changes in physical or dietary habits could indicate that the gut is not functioning well. An unexpected loss of weight can cause bacterial overgrowth in the small intestinal. Weight gain could be an indication that insulin resistance is present.

The previous section, we urged to make an outline of any your current health issues. Review this list right now. What percentage of these problems resemble the ones listed previously mentioned?

Habits that can harm the gut

There are a myriad of things we perform every day that result in bad gut health. Being aware of these behaviors is vital to implement changes in your daily routine that help you improve your health and wellbeing. Some habits seem to be harmless. If you don't know the ways these habits can affect your gut health it is possible to continue these habits that can cause uncomfortable discomfort and serious health issues that you might otherwise stay clear of.

Don't poo whenever you have to There are a variety of reasons to not be able to hold it in when must go. In the first place, if you don't eliminate waste from your body, it triggers the waste bi-products of the process to be absorbed by the body. The process of holding it in can cause constipation and make it difficult to get it out. The extra effort make in getting the stool out could lead to hemorrhoids developing because the veils surrounding the anus begin to expand. Intentionally putting your poop in the toilet can also result in your system becoming overloaded. If you're not getting rid of debris, it can cause impaction, in which the waste causes obstructions all the way to the digestive tract. There will be intense nausea and pain. When you notice an impaction it is essential to seek medical attention immediately to remove the obstruction.

In the end, if you're continuously waiting for your next meal it will alter the way that your digestive system functions and also the signals sent to your brain. In time, the process of holding your poop could result in the rectum awaiting until the next batch of waste is deposited before signalling the brain that it's time to be eliminated. If you decide to get rid of it to the bathroom, the muscles surrounding the rectum stay tight, which makes it painful and difficult to get rid of the waste.

* Consuming too many over-the-counter drugs: The over-the-counter pain medicine and non-

steroidal antiinflammatory medications (NSAID) alter the gut bacteria. It is crucial to be aware of this as people who suffer from digestive issues are frequently ordered or advised to take specific painkillers to reduce symptoms. The drugs, although they can ease discomfort and pain, can also aggravate digestive issues.

*Eating later or over the night eating late at night increases the risk of developing heartburn. This can alter the biochemical clock, which regulates appetite. If we alter the clock, various functions in the digestive tract are disrupted. There is a possibility that you don't make certain hormones when you need them for example, melatonin to assist in the process of bringing you to sleep.

Although you might not be able to stop eating late into the night Try to have your last meal to at least two hours prior to your time of bed. Beware of late-night snacks, that can cause problems for your stomach.

Do not eat foods that are high in fiber or probiotic-rich food items The goal is to consume at minimum 25 % of your fiber per day to ensure an ideal gut health, however the majority of us only get less than half of what we need. Fiber aids in the digestion process by helping move food through the digestive tract and also helps regulate the bowel movements.

• Not drinking enough water The digestive system depends on water to digest food, take in nutrients and then move food through different areas that comprise the GI tract. Drinking insufficient water can cause dehydration. When you're dehydrated, you're more likely to suffer from diarrhea.

* Consuming large portions We are advised to eat three meals per day, and to take three or two snacks to aid in surviving until our next meal. However, not all people gain from this plan of eating. If you have gastric reflux or bloating, it is possible that your symptoms diminish by eating smaller meals less frequently during the day.

Consuming too fast Consuming food too quickly may increase the chance of developing stomach ulcers and acid reflux. When you eat fast, you're more likely to swallow air, that travels down your stomach with your food. The excess air could result in more gas and constipation.

* Consuming too many alcohol drinks: Consuming alcohol frequently increases the chance of developing ulcers inside the stomach. They can hinder their being healed in a timely manner. Alcohol can cause stomach discomfort, which can lead to diarrhea. If you drink regularly, it is more probable that you will experience dehydration that increases the likelihood of constipation. If you drink more than two drinks of alcohol every day, this could affect your digestive tract. If you're not ready to quit drinking alcohol completely, give yourself two alcohol-free days per week. Additionally, make sure to drink glasses of red wine that can benefit digestive health due to the polyphenols found within red wines.

Chewing gum often If you chew gum, you inhale air that makes you feel more and feel more bloated. The artificial sweeteners found in gum can be harmful for gut health.

Smoking can cause harm to every organ in the body, which covers all that comprise the intestinal tract. Smoking decreases the amount oxygen in the body , which could kill gut bacteria. The chemicals in cigarettes cause the formation of a biofilm throughout the digestive tract, making it harder for food to pass through the digestive tract, for nutrients to be absorbed and enzymes to travel into the food and make it easier to break it down.

* Indulging in too much sugar If your diet is comprised of mostly processed food items, you're probably consuming large quantities of sugar. Food isn't the only area where added sugar is a major factor. Soda is among the most well-known drinks which contain a lot of sugar added. Sugar is a cause of imbalances and negative reactions in intestinal bacteria. Sugar that is refined, including high-fructose corn syrup, causes inflammation throughout the body, which increases the chance of developing various health issues including severe issues related to the digestive tract.

Don't get an colonoscopy: Women who are older than of 50 must undergo regular colonoscopies in order to detect colon cancer.

Unfortunately. People are often embarrassed having to undergo the procedure, and typically put off the procedure until they encounter problems that require one. Colon cancer may be present without displaying any symptoms, and a colonoscopy could detect it early before it grows or causes permanent damage.

• Not getting enough physical activity into your schedule as we age it is typical that our physical activity will decline. Women are more likely to avoid vigorous exercise because of the risk of injury because of an increase in osteoporosis risk. Seniors tend to reduce their physical exercise. There is a time where you're encouraged to slow down your pace and take a break. Being less active may raise the chance of developing various diseases and can also affect the digestive system. This is not helpful for who are older and require more medical procedures which require an increase in sleep and recovery. Joint replacement surgery for the hip is a frequent scenario, especially for women who are at a greater risk of developing osteoporosis. This type of surgery is vital, but the combination of additional mattress rest and medications to ease pain, result in a rise in constipation in the majority of women.

Insufficient sleep The lack of sleep can disrupt our circadian rhythm, or our biological clock. rhythm. This results in various systems and processes to be out of sync and perform badly. Sleeping in a bad way can also affect the production of hormones. This could have a negative impact on the way the digestive tract functions and negatively affects the gut bacteria.

Understanding the symptoms of a weakened digestive tract is the initial step to improve your overall health. Understanding the contributing factors to poor gut health, and the habits you could be engaging in that can cause digestive problems will be the second step. The new knowledge gained can be utilized to achieve better digestive health.

How well do you know Your Gut?

Examine the list of behaviors that we've just talked about and record the behaviors that you are exhibiting that are damaging your digestive system. After you have a list of behaviors, come up with at least one method to get rid of these habits.

For example:

If you're above 50 years old or suffer from multiple symptoms of disease, it's recommended to schedule an appointment with your physician to determine the cause behind the problems.

If you're frequent drinkers of soda during the course of your day, begin by replacing one drink with a bottle or a glass of water. In the ideal scenario, you'd like to stay clear of this however, even an incremental change could bring about positive changes.

Chapter 6: Digging Deeper: All About Gut Health

We briefly talked about the microorganisms in the digestive tract . Before you get scared, remember that none of the bacteria is harmful in particular in the case of the gut. Your digestive tract the home of both bad and good bacteria. While having a bit of both is necessary but when the bad bacteria begin to grow larger than the good, we are faced with a variety of health issues but many of these issues do not are related to the digestive system.

When you finish this chapter, you'll be able to appreciate the need for a healthy and balanced gut. As you'll discover, our health in the gut is often linked to the health of our other organs and systems such as the heart, brain, and even the skin. By gaining the knowledge you gain through this chapter, you'll be able to think differently and think more deeply about making the health of your gut a important priority.

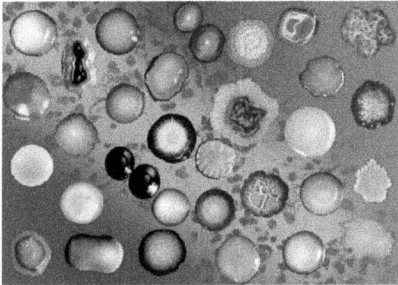

What exactly is Gut Health?

Gut health is the way the gastrointestinal tract performs. It is a consideration of how each part of the GI tract functions in conjunction with and independently of the other parts of the digestive tract. A healthy gut is unaffected of gastrointestinal symptoms and illnesses. A gut healthy indicates that all components that comprise the digestive tract work together while eating and throughout the digestion process. There shouldn't be any discomfort or pain as food is digested and processed.

In essence, gut health refers to development of bacterial colonies across all of the GI tract. Gut health is heavily influenced by the bacterial population. The diversity, quantity and function of these bacteria determines whether you're an unhealthy or healthy gut. Healthy guts will have an established microbiome. The microbiome is able to impact well-being in profound ways previously unnoticed.

What is the Gut Microbiome?

The term "gut microbiome" refers to the microorganisms in the intestinal tract. These microorganisms are comprised of the fungi, bacteria, and viruses. In the digestive tract, most of the microorganisms that are present are bacteria. One can have more than 1000 kinds of microbes or bacteria in the digestive system. If they are all combined, the microbes could weigh as much as 5 pounds. That's about the same as the brain's weight. They play a similar an important function.

The major portion of our gut bacterial is found in the large intestine , in the cecum or pocket of the intestines. There are a variety of bacteria found within the microbiome, and each one has a vital role to play in maintaining the health of our bodies to its best. The main function of these bacteria is to break down food items into vital nutrients. The bacteria that live within our gut are also responsible for transmitting and receiving signals from the brain.

Certain bacteria could cause harm if they are cultivated in excess. However, even the less-than-good bacteria are necessary to ensure a healthy environment for beneficial bacteria to flourish in. Gut microbes are vital to maintain the proper functioning of your body and good well-being. The gut must be stocked with various good bacteria that boost your immunity, decrease the symptoms associated with depression maintain your weight at a healthy level and also improve other aspects of your health. The microbiota in the gut is responsible to protect and defending the GI tract. They also play an important function in digestion and distribution of the essential nutrients that the body needs.

A diverse microbiome is essential. It means that a healthy and balanced microbiome must contain some bad bacteria as well as plenty of beneficial bacteria (which is also known by the name flora). Good bacteria require both insoluble and soluble fibers to feed off, and plenty of it. The bad bacteria thrive when we consume sugar or processed food items. The body is in a symbiotic relation to the microbiome. Microorganisms are absorbed then digested and converted into the compounds that your need for the body. This is why we require healthy and harmful bacteria.

How gut bacteria affect health

Gut bacteria play such an essential part in the body's processes and functions that without it we'd not be able to live. The gut bacteria we have growing alongside us over the past hundreds of years and due to this deep connected relationship, the microbes of our gut have learned to make sure that our body is in good health, ensuring that they have an environment in which to flourish.

From the moment you are born the gut microbiome active in regulating different processes and systems. It doesn't happen randomly as we direct influence the our gut bacteria through diet as well as other lifestyles. Our gut bacteria can affect the overall state of our health a few important ways.

The more different our gut bacteria, is the more beneficial for your health. The majority of our gut bacteria will interact with our body , where both the bacteria as well as the body are benefiting from their interaction. A few of the ways in which gut bacteria affect the body are:

* allowing us to digest the majority of food items we consume

* Producing enzymes which break down polysaccharides, or complex carbs.

* giving us B vitamins Vitamin K, short-chain acid fatty acids

The process of determining nutritional values for food

* helping to teach the immune systems that foreign invaders can be harmful or friendly

* stimulating the tissues in the gut to create antibodies as needed.

* making serotonin and also dopamine.

* impacting how the body reacts to anxiety and stress

* aiding in regulating the brain's chemical balance

* stopping toxins from getting into bloodstreams

* regulating metabolism

* storing nutrients for later use. utilized by other cells in the body

* helps reduce inflammation

* increasing the integrity of tissue

There are many bacteria that live happily within your digestive tract. While all bacteria exert an impact on the fundamental functions, some may also be detrimental to the body. Each person has their own microbes, and this particular combination is influenced through our actions, whether for good or bad.

Vitality of Gut Microbiota

Although the microbiome is a part of the organism in the digestive tract it is a part of many different organs, systems and even the human body across the body. If the gut is stocked with greater amounts of beneficial bacteria, our organs as well as the systems of the body are able to function correctly. If the gut has more than pathogenic microbes, our bodily mental and emotional health is at risk in many ways. The healthy gut bacteria will lead to better overall health. If the health of our gut isn't taken seriously this could cause impairment and lead to complications in important organs, such as the heart and brain. Gut health issues can also manifest itself in the form of different skin irritations. It is essential to comprehend the way that digestion influences the function of these organs as well as how to make sure that the health of our gut and other organs are in good health.

Brain Health

We discussed the brain-gut connection in the first chapter and the ways they mirror each other in different ways. It is now time to discuss further the ways that poor brain health could affect digestion and the gut's health may affect the functions of the brain.

Health of your gut is found to influence brain regions that are responsible for emotional behavior as well as other cognitive functions. Gut bacteria are believed have both a direct and indirect impact on the health of the brain. There are certain bacteria that reside in the gut that release neurotransmitters which are then sent into the brain. Neurotransmitters play a crucial part in regulating mood as well as combating mental health issues such as depression. People who have an unhealthful gut usually have an increased amount of bad bacteria, and tend to be suffering from mental disorders.

The gut is also linked to the brain via hundreds of nerves. Gut bacteria could influence the way messages are transmitted via these nerves. The gut and the brain connect with different systems in the body. Gut bacteria can disrupt other systems and, could, in turn, have an adverse effect on the brain's functioning.

There have been numerous studies that show that the on the microbiome of the gut that can affect specific cognitive issues. Numerous studies have shown that people who are suffering from anxiety or depression experience an improvement in their symptoms once they start taking probiotics (Mohajeri and colleagues. (2018)).

There is also additional research being conducted to show the connection of gut health to an increased risk of other cognitive ailments like dementia--Alzheimer's disease in particular. Alzheimer's patients have a smaller diversity of their microbiome, and it has been observed that the most prevalent kinds of good bacteria are not present in those suffering from Alzheimer's (Wanucha 2018). Although more research is needed however, studies have shown that, if gut flora is replenished, it will slow or slow the process that cognitive impairment is causing.

Heart Health

Research has shown that people with a diverse microbiome with more beneficial bacteria than bad bacteria are at a lower chance of suffering from heart disease. Bad bacteria can contribute to heart disease due to their ability to release harmful chemicals, which can increase the blockages in the arteries. In addition, gut bacteria that are unhealthy generate trimethylamine-N-oxide (TMAO). TMAO increases the likelihood of certain conditions that can cause heart disease. Numerous studies have shown that people who have high levels of TMAO are over 60% likely be suffering from a serious condition of the cardiovascular system (Healthy gut and a healthy heart? 2021).

Gut microbes can also affect other crucial factors that increase the risk of developing heart-related diseases. For those suffering from diabetes, for instance can have better control over level of blood sugar if they've taken a diet rich in fiber. Fiber promotes the development of certain bacteria which create short-chain fat acids. These acids regulate blood sugar levels and the blood pressure.

Skin Conditions

The gut microbiome is an essential role in maintaining good immune function. If the microbiome of the gut is altered, it may hinder the proper immune response. If your immune system isn't responding proactively to foreign invaders, either unknown or harmful, within the body, it can cause skin issues like:

* atopic dermatitis

* acne vulgaris

* dandruff

* psoriasis

* eczema

* skin cancer

The skin and the gut have their own microbiome and the skin is second only to the gut and having the most microbes that are found within the body. The gut and the skin have two-way communication that runs through the immune system. This line of communication works in the same way as the line of communication between the gut and brain.

Many studies have shown a connection between the health of your gut and the condition of your skin. For instance, studies regarding Celiac disease, where people have a severe intolerance to gluten, has shown that those with this condition are more prone to skin issues (De Pessemier 2021). Research also shows that when people modify their diet to cut out gluten the majority of skin problems such as rashes go away. If gluten was introduced back to their diet and the skin issues resurfaced.

Additionally, when the body is subjected to specific pathogens in the environment and pathogens, it could have an effect on the digestive. For instance, when you expose your skin in direct light, your skin absorbs vitamin D. Vitamin D circulates throughout the body, and when it reaches the gut , it supplies vital nutrients to bacteria in the gut. People who have enough exposure to the sun have a healthier gut microbiome.

We're just beginning to explore the way that gut microbiome influences our general health. The heart, the brain and skin are three of the primary organs that microbes from the gut affect. If you've struggled in your weight loss or have you been wondering why you're having trouble keeping your weight in a healthy way this chapter will give you the answer to your queries.

How well do you know Your Gut?

There's plenty you may not know about your microbiota of your gut. The microbiota is an amazing and intriguing eco system that is operating inside our bodies. Here are some fascinating facts that just make it more important to maintaining an optimal digestive system.

Each person's gut is different. While certain species of bacteria can be found in the digestive tract of most people however, the diversity and the amount of bacteria differ from person to.

Two identical twins who share more than 99% of the identical genes, will only share around 20 percent in their microbiomes (Benenden Health n.d.).

The baby begins to develop their gut bacteria, derived from the bacteria that are passed from mother to child through breast milk.

The number of bacteria in the gut microbiome than human cells in the rest of our body.

* The microbiome contains more diversity than the rainforest.

* Your gut has been transformed since you were born. At the time you were born,, you were surrounded by a plethora of bacteria in your gut. For the first seven years after birth , your microbiome of your gut is shaped by the place you live as well as the foods you consume and numerous other factors that affect your environment.

Gastroenterologists will determine if you are more likely to being overweight or lean by analyzing the bacteria in your gut.

Weight and More: Looking at the link between Gut Health and weight gain/loss

Statistics indicate that one out of four women are overweight and women are more likely to struggle with obesity that males (National Institute of Diabetes and Digestive and Kidney Diseases 2021). Women are in a higher risk of having difficulty losing weight and keeping a healthy weight, due to many reasons. If you're among those women, it's likely that you've tried a variety of weight loss and diet plans but with little results. Have you ever been pointed that your weight problems might be more related to your gut health and not your diet?

As we discussed in an earlier chapter, there's about 100 trillion bacteria in the intestines. The bacterium is in contact with the foods you eat and the different kinds of bacteria can affect how the food items are digested and utilized by your body.

Certain bacteria, such as Christensenellacae, are a popular species that is found in greater numbers in the gut of those who are healthy or slim. The obese have different types of bacteria, which tend to be more widespread and usually have a smaller population of Christensenllacae and, in some cases, none whatsoever. This implies that the different kinds of gut bacteria may have an impact on weight, and can provide us with a deeper understanding of the reasons why certain people have a harder time losing weight, while others seem to be naturally slim. This chapter focuses on the impact the gut bacteria play in influencing various aspects that influence weight loss or gain.

How Gut Bacteria Influences Weight

The microbiota play a part in the way food is processed, and could determine how many nutrients and calories are absorbed by our bodies. Gut bacteria can also influence the body's processes that affect the body's weight. The kind of bacteria and the diversity of bacteria present in the gut may change the way that our body stores fat as well as utilizes energy.

Gut microbiomes could create an inability to lose weight several ways. If there's a lot of bad bacteria in your gut, it could make certain food items more difficult to break into smaller pieces. For instance, starches can be much more challenging to digest, and the majority of bad bacteria are unable to access the complex calories that are found in certain starches. This causes extra calories being absorbed by the bloodstream, which are then saved as fat.

Factors that Influence Weight

There are many links to gut health as well as other factors which increase the likelihood of becoming obese. Blood pressure as well as inflammation levels, insulin levels as well as other variables that are a source of concern for people who are obese or overweight are all in one way or another controlled by the microbes in our gut. The gut bacteria contribute to the rate of metabolism that has an impact on our body weight. It is essential to comprehend how microbes influence different factors, in order to are aware of the best ways to take good care of the gut to ensure weight loss and better health.

Insulin Sensitivity

Some microbes could modify insulin sensitivity, which affects weight gain. Some bacteria could decrease levels of sugar released into bloodstreams because it consumes more before it is taken in by other cells of the body. If excessive sugar is released into bloodstreams, it could cause disruption to the process by which the body uses insulin to absorb glucose. Insulin resistance may occur when the body is not able to utilize insulin in a proper manner. Cells, muscles as well as other organs which depend on glucose as fuel aren't receiving the energy they require because the insulin isn't being utilized correctly. In excess blood glucose is converted to fat, which is stored to be used later on.

Metabolism

Gut bacteria diversity is vital to regulate metabolism. The term metabolism refers to the amount of energy that our body uses during the course of the day (energy refers to the calories consumed through drinks and foods). If your metabolism is low, the body won't burn enough energy, resulting in weight increase. If our metabolism is speedier, our body requires more energy, which means that our body will need more calories in order to function.

Inflammation

The gut bacteria are responsible for regulating the contents of the bloodstream as well as what gets transferred to the rest of the digestive tract to release. When dysbiosis , or an imbalance in the gut microbiota is present the immune system triggers an inflamatory response. This is because of low-quality bacteria producing more inflammatory and cytokines or allowing harmful substances to be introduced into the bloodstream, which the immune system could not recognize. If there is a higher level of cytokines within the body, it exposes us to chronic inflammation of a low-grade. The immune system then is called upon to be active for longer time, which can cause inflammation throughout our body. The low-grade inflammation is known to increase weight and is a frequent occurrence in obese people. Inflammation has also been associated with brain disorders like Alzheimer's disease . It is also more common among those with depression.

Blood Pressure

The high blood pressure common among those who are obese, however having high blood pressure could increase the likelihood of overweight. There's been an increase in the number of studies being conducted to study the impact our microbes can have on blood pressure. It was discovered that beneficial bacteria living in the gut can lower blood pressure due to its ability to enhance liver function (Kalaba 2021). Numerous studies have discovered an intriguing finding: altering the microbiome of the gut led to lower blood pressure for those in whom medication and lifestyle modifications were not effective.

Cholesterol Levels

Many have heard of bad cholesterol or low-density lipoprotein however, do you understand the role it plays in your body? We are aware that having a higher level of LDL can put you at risk of developing serious health issues such as stroke and heart attack. But, LDL is a molecule that helps detox fat-soluble substances from the liver. In small quantities, LDL cholesterol particles are essential to transport fats throughout the bloodstream. Since blood is a water-based substance the fat molecules require carriers to carry them from the stomach to other cells and muscles in the body. Without the cholesterol particles fats could separate from blood and raise the chance of blood clots, as well as obstructions to blood vessels.

Alongside carrying fats around your body LDL cholesterol also draw excess fat as well as substances that are associated with fat. These are transferred to the liver as the LDL molecules are able to release the excess substances back into the liver. These compounds are then passed through the detoxification process of the liver and are expelled by the kidneys as urine. They are then transported to the intestines where they will be eliminated through fecal matter.

An appropriate quantity of LDL cholesterol is actually helpful in removing excessive toxins from the bloodstream. These levels of cholesterol increase and cause negative consequences on the body's health when they are aiding in the inflammation response that is triggered by your immune system. Certain bacteria, such as gram-negative ones, generate an excess amount lipopolysaccharide (LPS) that escapes through the intestinal wall and then enter the bloodstream. In the process, LDL cholesterol levels increase to remove the LPS, which is thought to be a toxins by the immune system. However, it can also trigger an inflammation response.

If the gram-negative bacteria are more dominant than other beneficial bacteria in the body, levels of cholesterol are elevated, indicating inflammation within the body. What could cause this is a problem with the liver, and how as well when the body releases LDL. LDL is not released to transfer cholesterol to the cells whenever required because it could already be moving through bloodstream to collect LDS.

This can cause obstruction in the vessel , which can lead to a variety of cardiovascular problems.

Balancing Gut Bacteria to aid in Weight Loss

The microbiome of your gut can decide whether weight loss efforts is successful or not. People who have difficulty maintaining an ideal weight can be able to shed weight and maintain it through altering the microbiome of their gut. A number of studies confirm this. The research was demonstrated that people who were trying to shed weight following particular diet plans were able to shed more weight when certain kinds of bacteria were found in the digestive tract (Daley 2021).

Food choices and levels in physical exercise are two main factors that affect our gut bacteria , and consequently can affect our weight. The presence of specific gut bacteria, such as Akkermansia muciniphila, and Christensenella minuta have been found to help in losing weight. Akkermansia helps to strengthen the intestinal lining. They create short chain fatty acids, which control the body's fat.

People who are slimmer or healthier tend to have greater amounts of these bacteria in their microbiome of their gut. You can boost the level of Akkermansia by incorporating certain food items into your diet.

* cranberries

* grapes

* rhubarb extract

* bamboo shoots

* black tea

* Fish oil

* Flaxseeds

Christensenella isn't found in the gut microbiome because it is linked to your genetic make-up. Families with members who have this kind of bacteria have a higher chance to be affected. If you don't have this type of bacteria it's not a problem. There are other kinds of bacteria can assist you to keep a healthy weight and even helping to prevent weight gain and other health problems that can be caused by excessive weight.

A different kind of bacteria may aid in the loss of weight Prevotella. Research has shown that this particular strain of bacteria can grow rapidly when fed fighting fuels. When Prevotelladigests food, it is likely to absorb more nutrients to use to use for their own. The same nutrients, if over-absorbed in bloodstreams will be converted into fat to fat and stored in the body.

Although your gut bacteria may remove excess fat or lead to reduction in weight but it does indirectly influences the weight. A diet rich in fiber is among the top suggested ways to promote the growth of healthy bacteria, which can result in greater weight control. Plant-based diets are also helpful in increasing the diversity of your microbiome.

Dieting is the Gut and Weight loss

If you're trying to shed some weight, you may be thinking about beginning a diet plan to assist you in achieving your weight reduction goals. It's important to point out that a lot of popular or popular diets could be bad for your gut health and general health. Many diets claim quick results but they're not always lasting or lasting outcomes. A lot of fad diets do not consider the negative effect of eliminating certain food groups, such as carbohydrates, or limiting the intake of food can have on your digestive tract.

There are a variety of reasons that diets are not effective to maintain weight loss over the long term. They can even increase the chance of further weight gain. This is the reason it is crucial to know how certain diets affect gut bacteria. The diets that advise that you should eliminate certain food groups could create changes in the gut microbiome but this won't necessarily benefit you in the long run.

Low-carb, high-fat diets like the ketogenic diet is an instance. The ketogenic diet encourages large amounts of fat consumption, while removing carbohydrates, especially ones from grains and fruits. These are the most important sources of fiber that nourish the gut microbiome. Research has proven that eating an excessive amount of fat and reducing the amount of fiber you would do on the Keto diet can reduce diversity of the gut microbiome (Yokoyama 2019,). In addition, low-fiber diets result in the bacteria in the gut not producing short-chain fatty acids, which help in reducing inflammation.

It's not necessary to follow the latest trending diet to keep your weight or gut health! Research has shown that people who ate a lot of plant-based food improved blood sugar levels as well as enhanced the growth of beneficial bacteria within the gut (Edermaniger 2020). Gut bacteria that are beneficial to us thrive on plant-based food as they supply our bodies various minerals and nutrients that gut bacteria eat. For instance, many fruit and vegetables are rich in of fiber, which will not only nourish our good bacteria but also aid in weight loss.

Consuming plant-based foods doesn't have to be complicated. It is not necessary to follow strict guidelines or rules as are typically the case when you follow the latest diet trend. Instead, you concentrate on being more aware of your food choices and take the decision to select foods from plants. This includes:

* fruits

* vegetables

* Whole grains

* lentils and beans

* seeds and nuts

* Tofu

* tempeh

* vegetable oils (extra virgin olive oil, avocado oil, sesame oil)

Although you would like a large portion of your meals to be comprised of plant-based ingredients, it does not mean that you must or desire to eliminate other food categories. Fish that contain omega-3s such as salmon, sardines and tuna is beneficial to brain health. We all know that when our brains are in good health, our digestive system will reflect this healthy state. Lean protein from food sources provides your body amino acids which help create proteins in our bodies.

When you change to a vegan diet, you'll notice that your digestion will naturally improve. Just add more vegetables into your meals, as well as opt for fresh vegetables and fruits as snacks. These two small changes can make a significant impact on your overall well-being.

After having learned how gut microbiota influences weight gain then it's time to find out how you can gain better control over your gut well-being by encouraging a diverse and healthy microbiome in your gut. We have already mentioned that the consumption of plant-based foods is highly advised, in the following section you will be taught about specific varieties of foods that change the gut microbiome positively.

How well do you know Your Gut?

The microbes that live in your gut could aid you in maintaining your body's form and help explain why certain people are more secure against obesity and weight gain. After you've figured out the crucial role that the microbiota of your gut is playing in influencing weight gain It is the right time to understand the ways that your gut bacteria might be hindering your efforts to lose weight.

Begin to keep track of your food and drinks regularly. Be honest about your tracking. There is no need to keep track of calories or the amount you consumed. Make a note of all the foods you consume. Keep this list for a few days and you'll be able to realize why this is beneficial in the coming chapters.

Chapter 7: Food For The Gut: What To Eat For A Healthy Gi

Did you catch Chelsea's story from our introduction? She was able to get rid from the ruthless dieting cycle and notice a dramatic improvement in her health and weight after seeking assistance from an expert in nutrition. With the assistance of her nutritionist Chelsea could develop an approach that was focused on improving her digestion. The weight gradually began to fall off. Her digestive problems she was struggling to deal with each day ended up being a thing of past. Her overall health was improved dramatically.

Making a plan to heal your gut is to identify the foods that are best for your digestive tract (GI). By having this list you'll know what foods you should have at home. It will also identify the food items that cause digestive problems and then eliminate them from your kitchen to avoid the temptation. Furthermore, Chelsea found great reliance in preparing specific menus that helped her learn how cook in a healthy gut method. The meals she cooked were, to her delight, were not boring or boring.

It is possible that you have the same idea that Chelsea first had. Healthy food is bland and ineffective. But this isn't the reality. You can make tasty meals that are healthy and will keep your family returning for more. When Chelsea realized how easy it was to make an eating plan, she started using it on a regular basis in her home . It was beneficial to her as well as the whole family.

When you are aware of what foods are beneficial in your digestion, you are able to start to make better diet choices. It will also help you identify which foods to eliminate or reduce your intake to ensure good gut health. However, this doesn't mean you must adhere to strict guidelines regarding what you should and shouldn't consume. What you will find is the fact that there's plenty of options of foods which will help you increase your health and lose weight without feeling overwhelmed. When you are done with this chapter, you'll be able to see that you don't need to complicate your food plans or be overwhelmed by thinking about which food choices are most beneficial to your overall health.

The Best Food Types for better Gut Health

Certain foods can help maintain your gut health and help you lose weight. Certain foods can aid in the absorption of nutrients, and help keep the gut microbiome in balance and healthy. Keep in mind that the microbiota of your gut is a dynamic environment and the different types of bacteria will require a diverse variety of nutrients in order to thrive.

The most effective way to ensure the health of your gut and to promote an array of beneficial gut microbiomes is to eat a diverse variety of plant-based food (as we have discussed earlier in this chapter). Ensure that you have enough nutrition and vitamins will ensure that your gut microbes are healthy. The most important food sources to incorporate into your balanced diet are listed below.

High-Fiber Foods

Fiber-rich foods help keep our guts healthy due to a variety of reasons. They nourish the gut bacteria through prebiotics and other nutrients that healthy gut flora needs to thrive. While the body isn't able to process fiber, gut bacteria are able to. If they do, they help to promote an array of microbes that can help you maintain the weight you need to be at. A few studies have revealed that those who consumed fruit and vegetables rich in fiber could stop the growth of intestinal bacteria that are known to cause an increase in likelihood of contracting certain diseases (Robertson 2021).

Certain high-fiber food items like artichokes, apples, almonds and even artichokes can boost the growth rate of the Bifidobacterial bacteria. The Bifidobacterium has been proven to lower inflammation in the intestines and aids in maintaining good gut health. Other foods rich in fiber that can benefit your health include:

* Whole grain

* legumes

* Beans

* pea

* Oats

* Banana

* berries

* asparagus

* leeks

Fermented Foods

In the process of fermentation, the sugars present in the food are broken into smaller pieces by bacteria or yeast. These foods act as probiotics which is live microorganisms that can be extremely beneficial to the gut health when eaten.

Fermented foods also contain lactobacilli , which helps improve the health of your gut. It has also been proven that those who consume foods that contain lactobacilli have a lower level of certain harmful bacteria, such as Enterobacteriaceae that can trigger inflammation within the body.

Fermented foods can help boost the development of good bacteria and enhance the function of bacteria within the digestive tract. People who experience frequent diarrhea may benefit from balancing their gut by taking probiotics found in fermented food items to ease these digestion issues.

Examples of foods that are fermented include:

* Kimchi

* sauerkraut

* yogurt

* tempeh

* miso

* Kefir

Many people opt for yogurt to maintain a healthy digestive system and it is recommended to help promote healthy growth of bacterial species in the digestive tract. But, you must be aware of the kind of yogurt you pick. A majority of yogurts that are flavored contain high levels of sugar that could limit the benefits you can get from eating yogurt. When you are choosing

140

foods that contain fermented ingredients such as yogurt, be sure to be sure to read the labels before you purchase. Look for products that claim "contains active cultures that live" to reap the maximum benefits.

Polyphenol-Rich Foods

Polyphenols are plant-based compounds which have numerous positive effects on general health. The body is unable to process many polyphenols, but they are essential for the gut bacteria. They also reduce the level of triglycerides as well as C-reactive proteins, both which can cause inflammation in the body.

Best polyphenol-rich foods include:

* dark chocolate

* Green tea

* Red wine

* grape skins

* Almonds

* Onions

* blueberries

* Broccoli

Many polyphenols encourage the growth of beneficial bacteria and reduce the number of bad bacteria. For instance, cacao or dark chocolate can increase Bifidobacterium as well as Lactobacilli. However, at the same time Clostridia development slows down.

Collagen-Boosting Foods

Collagen is commonly considered to be an ingredient that can help improve hair, skin and nails. Collagen is an amino acid found naturally in our bodies and is utilized to build connective tissue throughout. Our ligaments, tendons bones, skin and our guts all depend on collagen for the proper shape and functioning. In the gut area, it is important to note that collagen could assist in the repair of injuries that is caused by inflammation. It can also defend the gut from harm.

It's easy to locate collagen supplements almost everywhere, even though they are usually advertised for better hair and skin. It is important to be careful when purchasing collagen supplements. There are numerous types of collagen supplements, and not all can be absorbed easily into the body. Large collagen molecules can require a longer time to digest and collagen molecules might not be fully taken in. The hydrolyzed collagen supplements are decreased to a smaller size for the digestive tract, but they are processed in excess and are of low quality.

You can consume collagen via our diet. The most effective sources of collagen-rich foods are:

* Bone broth

* Salmon

* mushrooms

Foods to avoid

Be aware that the food we consume can either fuel the good bacteria or feed the bad bacteria. It isn't enough to consume more of the food items that help the beneficial bacteria. You must remove or reduce your intake of food items that feed the bad bacteria. Simply eating more foods that are rich in fiber and drinking a liter of soda every day, will not alter the microbiota of your gut in the way you want. To maintain your health in the gut, you need to ensure that good bacteria have enough nutrition to thrive, and also eliminate those that are harmful to your gut. The food items listed here will not be a shock to you however, studies have only just discovered the specific issues they create for your gut health.

Artificial Sweeteners

Artificial sweeteners such sucrallose or aspartame, are popular sugar substitutes people who want to shed weight will use. They have no calories and contain no sugar, which can lead to the impression that they're beneficial to your health. Artificial sweeteners do not get absorbed by the body, but once they come into contact with bacteria in the gut, they are rapidly consumed. They have a negative effect on the gut bacteria as well as altering the microbiome. The altered gut bacteria can increase the likelihood of having glucose intolerance.

A majority of us consume an excessive amount of sugar added and artificial sweeteners every day. The processed sugar depletes the good flora that lives in our guts and fuels the harmful. If we starve the good plants of nutrition, it will die but initially, they'll attempt to live by feeding on the lining of our intestinal tract, which results in an rise in inflammation.

Beware of artificial sweeteners that are frequently utilized in diet products. Foods advertised as being low-calorie usually include some or all artificial sweeteners. This is a common feature in food items, such as yogurt, which you'd think would improve your digestion. It is essential to read the label of any products you buy and to learn how to spot artificial sweetener ingredients that may be found in a variety of common foods you consume.

Foods processed for processing

Foods processed for processing lack essential nutrients, particularly beneficial ones such as fiber. Many processed foods contain greater quantities of sugar as well as salt and artificial ingredients. Microbiomes that are unhealthy thrive on these ingredients, but healthy microbes need a range of nutritious, fibrous and nutrient-rich food items.

Processed food is all foods that have been through a process where nutrients are removed from their natural sources. This includes the majority of sweets and snacks and also a variety of prepackaged food items, such as the white flour as well as table sugar. While many people love these food items but it is highly advised to limit the amount you consume.

The most effective way to reduce the amount of processed food is to concentrate on eating a wide variety of colourful foods, including vegetables and fruits. Another suggestion is to start making some meals and snacks in order to reduce the amount of snacks you consume during the day, and replace the unhealthy options with healthier ones.

Red Meat

Carnitine is a component of red meats that encourages the release trimethylamine Noxide upon processing through certain bacteria in the gut. We've discussed TMAO in the past and how it can contribute to the build-up of plaque within the arterial. The research suggests a clear correlation with the gut microbiome's interaction with red meats, and an rise in serious health issues like heart disease.

While you require some of the fatty acids that red meats provide but you should restrict your consumption in order to keep your gut healthy. As opposed to red meats opt for the fatty fish and plant-based proteins like beans and tofu in order to obtain the ideal amount of nutrients to keep your gut and its bacteria healthy.

Food has the greatest impact on your gut health since it is the primary factor that promotes the development of either good or bad bacteria. However, it isn't the only thing you need to be aware of. When you have addressed your diet and decide to eat more proper foods, there are couple of other strategies you can use to improve your digestive tract.

How well do you know Your Gut?

Then, at the end of the chapter that you were asked to keep track of every meal and drink you consumed for a couple of days. Review your journal now and see how many items you have listed fall in the "foods to consume" category, and what percentage fall into the "foods to stay clear of" category? Don't be embarrassed if you find yourself eating more of the items to stay clear of compared to suggested foods. But, it is important to look at your food diary and determine how you can incorporate more of the food items that contribute to greater gut health.

If you've not kept track of your food intake You can start tracking your food today. Check your fridge and pantry right today. What are the most common items you have in your kitchen that are on the recommended food list? Are you able to make meals with only the items recommended for the coming day, or two days? If not, take a few minutes and write a list of grocery items of the items you'll have to purchase at the market.

No Guts and No Glory Tips to Get an Optimal GI

Do you realize that having dirty teeth can cause stomach problems? Keep in mind that the mouth is an integral part of the digestive tract (GI). According to research, the inability to wash your teeth properly could result in the development of billions of harmful bacteria that could get into your gut and trigger inflammation (Van Hare 2017). From our teeth to sleep , and all the things between, the gut health is affected by numerous aspects.

It is possible that as you make changes to your diet and lifestyle, your digestive system may not be as open to the modifications. For many, removing digestive problems, improving overall health, and losing weight, requires taking into consideration the various elements of an ideal way of life. A commitment to a healthy life at any age is the most effective option to guarantee healthier health.

Strategies to Improve Gut

Food is an essential ingredient to maintain a healthy digestive system living a healthy and balanced way of life is equally important. A more healthy way of life that focuses on improving every aspect of your mental and physical health can help your gut in many ways. When you are able to implement healthy lifestyle changes , one at each step, you'll feel better and see that these little changes improve your weight.

Dental Hygiene

Rememberthat your mouth is your first point of entry for food during the digestion process. A lot of people aren't aware of how their dental health may negatively impact your gut's health. Gut health is a matter of proper dental hygiene.

In the mouth, bacteria can be transported to the gut to alter the bacteria. The gut bacteria aren't very friendly to the bacteria that are invading their territory. Oral bacteria can also be responsible for causing various stomach-related issues and increasing the likelihood of developing IBD. (IBD). In addition, the buildup of oral bacteria causes an immune response which could lead to the an enlargement of the stomach.

If you have dental health issues, this could cause problems with nutrient absorption. One of the initial signs of a poor gut condition is usually discovered through dental issues. Gingivitis or bleeding on the gums is an indication of inflammation that may affect other components in your digestive tract. The most common symptoms you could notice in your mouth that could suggest poor health in your gut include:

* Red patches that are flat on the gums, or on the inside of the cheeks. They are often lesions that occur because of the vitamin B12 deficiency. The digestive tract might not absorb this vitamin in a proper manner or you might not be getting enough of it in your diet. Inflammatory digestive conditions such as Crohn's disease and atrophic gastritis may hinder the the proper intake of vitamin B12

* Oral candida Oral candida: This is an infection , which typically is the result of an imbalance in the immune system. It could also arise because of zinc deficiency. If you are on antibiotics, take a large amount of sugar, have a baby or

identified with diabetes mellitus it is more probable that you will develop oral candida. The most common sign of the condition is a swelling of the tongue, which is red.

• Mouth ulcers. Ulcers that occur in the mouth may be caused by inflammation and red gums. These signs could indicate an imbalance in the immune system.

The burning mouth disorder results in an intense burning sensation in your mouth. There is also a losing taste swelling, as well as dry and dry mouth. If these symptoms are present typically, it's an indication that you are not receiving enough vitamins or minerals. If you are taking an antidepressant medication, that medication could also cause similar symptoms.

It is essential to ensure that you make good dental hygiene a top priority. Regularly brushing, flossing, and rinsing your mouth regularly with mouthwash is a great way to keep your mouth healthy. Plan regular visits to the dentist for thorough cleanings is highly recommended to maintain your gut and your mouth well.

Exercise

Exercise is essential to improve overall health. While most people are aware that they need to exercise regularly to keep their heart well-maintained and maintain a healthy weight, not many realize how vital it is for the gut health. Exercise is a natural way to reduce stress levels, which can help in warding away inflammation. Regular exercise is also proven to have an impact on the gut microbiome.

Regular exercisers are found to have a larger diversity of microbiome. Numerous studies have demonstrated that professional athletes carry more Akkermansiaceae bacteria that are known to decrease the risk of being overweight (Beil and Cherry, 2019,). It doesn't mean you should start working out as the Olympian athlete. A study that looked at how exercise impacts gut bacteria revealed that people who completed a 30 minute workoutthree times per week, experienced an increase in gut flora in only six weeks (Well+Good Editors, 2019,).

A small increase in your physical activity will help maintain a healthy digestive system.

Activities that require minimal effort can ease numerous digestive issues. The slight increase in movement assists in the movement of waste and food into the digestive tract. this is particularly beneficial for those who suffer from constipation. A low-impact, light intensity exercises that you can start include:

* Walking

* Cycling

* Yoga

* abdominal exercises, such as abdominal crunches or sit-ups

* Tai Chi

While keeping to a moderate intensity workout such as the ones listed above are great but it's not unwise to incorporate an hour or two of intense interval training (HIIT). These kinds of exercises raise the heart rate up and maintain it even after the exercise is completed. They also provide the immune system an increase in performance since the body is likely to experience some slight increases in inflammation.

If you're experiencing any GI issues , it is best to avoid high-impact training that is low-intensity and low-impact. Although a slight increased inflammation could help to strengthen your immune system, this could create more issues with your digestive system. In addition it is true that HIIT exercises shift circulation from your GI system to muscles to help you perform your exercise with a high intensity. The decreased flow of blood to the gut slows the digestion system, which may cause constipation as well as other stomach-related discomforts.

Stress Management

Stress is a normal state that we encounter at different times throughout the day. While a tiny amount of stress will not be enough to cause major gut problems, prolonged stress can have a negative impact on your health. In terms of the health of your gut, stress may result in a number of problems. The high levels of cortisol (the cortisol hormone that is associated with stress) causes inflammation. As we've mentioned before inflammation can cause damage to different parts of the digestive tract, and raise the chance of developing autoimmune diseases.

Stress can also increase our desire for carbs and sugars. The reason for this is the fact that stress causes the body to go into fight or flight mode. If this occurs the brain automatically emits signals to signal that it is in need of fuel in order to fight an opponent or avoid the perceived threat. It doesn't matter if you're actually in danger of imminent harm. The body is unable to determine between a potentially life-threatening situation (which will require more energy to get through) or a situation that is less urgent (such as a jam in the traffic which makes you late for work). Stress even in small amounts can cause disruption to the digestive tract.

It is essential to begin to adopt effective techniques for managing stress which will assist you in battling anxiety on a daily basis. The most recommended methods to manage stress include:

* Mediation

* massages

* exercise

* journaling

* Yoga

* spending time with your loved ones

* Take a walk in the nature

* reduce caffeine intake

* Aromatherapy

* cuddle your pet

Engaging in one stress-reducing activity each day can help maintain stress levels at an acceptable level. It is equally important to understand how to manage anxiety all day. Simple mindfulness exercises will instantly lower the stress levels down. Breathing deeply for long periods of time while exhaling slowly is an additional technique to manage stress at the present.

Sleep

If we don't get enough rest, our digestive tract becomes out of the rhythm of its natural processes. The digestion process can occur as the digestive tract is meant to relax and making use of less energy. Inability to adhere to a regular sleeping schedule could cause disruption to the production of hormones, including the appetite suppressant and hunger hormones that can cause an increase in weight-related issues and other health problems.

In addition, when we're tired, we may crave more sweet food items. This is due to our body telling us that we require more energy to make it through the day. If we mix the increased craving for sugar along with our knowledge that we tend to make bad eating choices, it's an ideal recipe for a sluggish digestive system.

To make sleeping an important thing, make sure you create a space that encourages sleep. If you are a habitual user of the TV on until you're unable to focus your eyes any further, shut it off before you go to sleep. Avoid all electronic devices for at least a half hour before going to the time you go to bed, to allow your mind a chance to unwind.

Below is some recommendations to think about that could aid in promoting sleep.

* Turn the temperature of your bedroom to 68 degrees.

* Apply aromatherapy, like lavender sprays or incense, to calm your mind and body.

* Choose tranquil and relaxing activities before bedtime, like writing or reading.

* Try to sit for five minutes prior to getting to bed.

* Include the five minutes of yoga routine to help you get sleeping.

* Make sure to have the proper sheets, blankets and pillows on your mattress. Also , make sure that they are cleaned or changed every week at least.

• Maintain the ventilation in your bedroom.

Do not drink anything within an hour or less prior to the time you go to bed.

Beware of napping throughout the day, or limit the length of naps to 60 minutes.

Stop your caffeine consumption before 2 pm.

* Try to fall asleep at the same time each night.

Your bedroom should be kept to only sleeping.

* Take a strenuous walk between two and three hours prior to the time you have set for time for bed.

Be aware of the humidity levels. Insufficient humidity in the air could cause mold to float about , making breathing difficult throughout the night.

Use a sound device to help you fall asleep. sleep.

* Use an eye mask If your partner would prefer to scroll through their smartphone or browse their iPad rather than sleep.

If you're having trouble falling asleep and you are struggling to fall asleep, don't force yourself to stay awake shifting and tossing. Instead, it's best to get up and engage in a peaceful and quiet task like such as a term search, reading or even journaling. Make sure to not turn on the lights or use warm-toned lighting so that you don't trigger brain's waves. When you start to get tired, go back to your bed.

It is crucial to make an effort to enjoy a full night of restful sleep. If you notice that going into a good sleep for the duration of all night seems to be a frequent problem for you, talk to your physician. It could be beneficial to have sleep studies that could pinpoint the root of your difficulties in getting a good night's sleep.

Slow Down Food When You Eat

Making sure you chew your food thoroughly and taking time to savor your food can help you combat common digestive problems. Fast eating can result in taking in more air when you eat, which could cause you to experience more bloating as well as abdominal pain. If you do not chew your food correctly, it could be difficult for your digestion tract to break down the food into smaller pieces, which means your body won't get all the vitamins and nutrients it requires from the food we consume.

To slow down the pace of eating when you eat Try sitting down during your meal. We tend to hurry even more when we're grabbing things on the go, or while running around. Consider incorporating conscious eating or intuitive eating methods. They are two eating habits that require slowing down and paying attention to the food you consume. They can help bring greater attention to the food you eat to help you enjoy the food you eat more. When you eat, pay attention into aspects of your meal. Take a moment before you put that first taste of food into your mouth, and observe the smell and appearance of your food. When you eat your food, take a break from the process of chewing so that you can enjoy the flavor and taste, as well as the texture and the way the tongue feels. It is not necessary to pay attention to every bite but taking a moment to pause each bite and incorporating your other senses to your food can help you to slow down when you eat.

Hydration

Drinking enough water is vital to combating constipation. However, there are many other reasons to drink enough water to keep our guts well and healthy. Drinking enough water helps keep the mucosal lining of intestinal tract lubricated, allowing them to perform their tasks effectively. Water also aids to keep the healthy bacteria that live in our guts healthy and balanced.

It is suggested that you consume half your daily weight in ounces. If you weigh 170 pounds , you must aim to drink 85 ounces of fluids each every day. It may feel like an excessive amount of water, particularly if you're not regularly having water in the morning. To boost your intake of water, consider these suggestions:

Drink a glass of cold water the moment you get up at dawn. This will not only help you rehydrate after a night of sitting and sleeping, but it can also stimulate the digestive tract to awaken and get active.

* Drink an ounce of water prior to when eating. Drinking plenty of water prior to a large meal can aid your digestive tract in breaking down

163

food properly and decrease the chance of eating too much.

* Keep a water bottle at the place where in the areas where you spend in the majority of your day. You'll be more likely to grab an ounce of water at work when it is easily accessible. A bottle of water at hand will lessen the urge to pull over and take a drink while you go on around on your errands.

* Flavor your water. Utilize fresh fruits like strawberries, kiwi, or watermelon for a refreshing change. Drinking water that is plain can be boring for many, therefore having a few ideas to spice up your drink with some additional flavor can help you meet that daily goals.

* Remember to get a boost in water from the foods you consume. Cucumbers or watermelon, as well as celery are fantastic snacks that can keep you well-hydrated throughout the day.

Food Intolerances

It's not unusual for people to not be aware of food intolerances since the symptoms might not be constant or they may not be aware that the symptoms they feel are related to the food they consume. Food intolerance can lead to various symptoms, including:

* cramping

* Bloating

* stomach pains

* diarrhea

* Rash

* nausea

* fatigue

* acid reflux

Eggs, gluten, dairy yeast, nuts and caffeine are a few of the most frequent food intolerances that sufferers struggle with. If you have any of the symptoms mentioned above, start to monitor your symptoms and the foods you consume. There could be a pattern that seems to that shows symptoms becoming more frequent after eating certain trigger food items. It is also possible eliminating common trigger foods like whole wheat, milk, coffee, and rye that could help reduce symptoms of food intolerance.

If you find that your digestive discomfort diminishes after you have stopped eating these trigger foods, it is advisable to think about changing your diet. It is possible to continue eating certain foods, however in smaller amounts. If removing these foods isn't enough to be helping the digestive issues you are experiencing, check with your doctor to determine what other foods are creating problems for you.

Vitamins, supplements, and Pro/Prebiotics

The use of supplements and vitamins will increase your intake of specific minerals and nutrients that you might not get enough from your diet alone. The beneficial vitamins you should think about taking to improve your digestive health include:

* vitamin A

* vitamin B12

* vitamin C

Vitamin D

* iron

* Selenium

* zinc

Prebiotics and prebiotics can be extremely beneficial in improving the health of your digestive system. Prebiotics feed the gut bacteria, and also encourage the growth of beneficial bacteria. These live microbes help replenish good bacteria that could be destroyed by having an antibiotic or a serious illness. Certain foods can act as prebiotics, for example:

* legumes

* Oats

* bananas

* Garlic

* asparagus

Certain foods be probiotics, such as:

* yogurt

* fermented food items

* bread made from sourdough

* miso

You may also decide to consume prebiotic or probiotic supplements. Be aware that some prebiotics and probiotics are of top quality and could cause greater harm than beneficial. The same is true for all other vitamins and supplements too. It is recommended to consult with your physician to help you choose the highest quality supplements to boost the health of your gut.

If you're planning on getting an additional fiber to ease your digestive problems, you should know there are a variety of digestive problems result from lack of fiber. Women can experience digestive issues due to a drop in of the pelvic floor or in weakening. A lot of women use supplements with fiber when they suffer with digestive issues such as constipation however this could cause symptoms of weak pelvic floors worse. It is crucial to talk to your doctor to rule out any other conditions which could trigger digestive issues prior to taking any supplements.

The Gut Health Issues

What happens if you're doing everything correctly but have a problem with your digestion problems? When is the right time to bring problems with digestion with your physician? It's easy to dismiss digestive problems or misinterpret them for common aches. If you're suffering from discomfort or have stomach issues often or frequently, these could be a sign of serious illnesses. All chronic digestive problems should discuss the issue with a physician. The following signs should prompt you to consult a physician:

* chronic abdominal discomfort

* persistent and severe heartburn

Trouble swallowing

* pain in swallowing

* frequent sore throats or hoarseness

Feeling like you've got some kind of thing stuck to your chest or throat

* episodes of choking

169

* nausea or vomiting that won't stop

* constipation or chronic diarrhea

* Blood in stool or stool that is dark in color

* Loss of appetite

Unexplained weight loss

* persistent gas, bloating, or gas

If you've been making lifestyle changes and are able to honestly alter your diet to improve digestion, your digestive problems will lessen or cease completely. Although most digestive issues will improve by themselves However, some may require additional assessment to ensure the right treatment. It is recommended to consult your physician if you experience digestive problems no matter if they are mild or severe.

Make sure to schedule regular checks that are related directly on you GI tract. Over 50s should undergo annual colonoscopies. However, if you're in good health, you might be in a position to wait until 60 or more to think about regular testing for cancer.

Now you understand the crucial influence our digestive system plays on general health. You are aware of how our digestive system affects our weight and could result in other health issues that are typically thought to not be related to the health of our gastrointestinal system. Although you have learned a myriad of ways to maintain an ideal gut, you might have a few questions that you want to answer in order to help you create an action plan. This chapter is going to take off any questions you may have lingering about your gut.

How well do you know Your Gut?

You've read a few of suggestions that could affect the health of your digestive system. What other elements do you use? What do you think can be changed? What are the best habits to adopt in order to get to your an optimal state of health?

Write down the actions you think you'll must tackle in order to better your overall health.

Select one exercise to begin with, and then create a second list of tasks you can begin doing to begin creating a healthy routine.

For example, you might realize that your main issue is getting enough sleep. Are you able to begin making a an inventory of the things you can do to make you be less stressed at the end of the day? Do you have the ability to adopt better habits that will assist you in falling asleep and sleep through the night?

Make the effort to adopt changes gradually. Follow the guidelines in this chapter to provide a foundation to help you begin making changes to your everyday life. After you've successfully adopted the one habit you want to change, you can move to the next. In order to achieve optimal gut health, it is recommended to incorporate all one of the healthy living habits.

Chapter 8: Questions About Gut Health

This chapter is designed to ensure that you complete the book with all the knowledge as you require about the health of your gut and its relationship in weight loss. In contrast to the earlier chapters, which sought to provide comprehensive coverage of all factors of gut health and weight loss, Chapter 8 will give you the most frequently asked questions and answers regarding the health of your gut. After this chapter, will feel more confident in making the small , but effective adjustments that are required for getting the results you want.

How does coffee affect gut Health?

Coffee has a negative as well as positive effect on gut health. Coffee contains soluble fiber that helps to feed the good bacteria within the gut. A small cup of coffee at midday is not likely to cause digestive problems. But, caffeine content in coffee may cause problems. Also the addition of sugar, milk or even cream could decrease the amount of fiber in your coffee since the sugar and milk nourish the undesirable microbes in your gut.

What is the effect of Alcohol affect the health of your gut?

Alcoholic beverages may affect several areas within the GI tract. The most frequent and worrying issues are:

* loss of enamel on teeth, leading to an increase in the development of cavities

* increased risk of disease in the gums and gum infections

* higher risk of developing the gastroesophageal reflux disorder (GORD)

* heartburn that is more frequent

* damage to the liver that can result in cirrhosis. In this case, the liver is unable to function normally.

* Small intestinal bacterial growth (SIBO) that causes constipation, cramps, excessive gas and diarrhea

* Pancreas damage that affects insulin production and impairs the function of digestive enzymes.

* irritation of the mucosa of the intestine

* harmful changes to microbiota in the gut and a decrease in the diversity of gut bacteria

• weight loss, particularly around the abdomen.

Women are at greater chance of developing digestive problems due to the consumption of alcohol. Female livers are 30 percent smaller than the male liver, which makes it more difficult to process alcohol (Ryan and McGowan 2021). People who were diagnosed IBS or are suspecting they be suffering from the disease will notice that their symptoms get worse. Women are also at a higher risk of being diagnosed IBS and the increasing difficulty to detoxify alcohol, the consumption of alcohol can be a problem.

Although you don't have to stop drinking alcohol completely however, it is important to drink with a sense of responsibility. Limit your drinking to just one or two drinks. Always drink a glass of water after every drink and try not to drink with a full stomach.

What are the effects of certain medications on the health of your gut?

Numerous medications can alter the microbiome in the gut. These include painkillers (as previously discussed within this publication) along with laxatives, antihistamines and female hormones like estrogen that are taken during menopausal cycles. In addition, medications can create imbalances in the microbiota of the gut and can cause irritation to the mucosa of the intestinal.

Certain medications do not affect the gut bacteria in the same manner. Certain drugs can kill the gut bacteria and others may decrease diversity, and some slow the development of beneficial bacteria. In addition to the mediation that we've previously discussed throughout the book, there are also medicines to avoid:

* Blood pressure medication

* cholesterol-lowering medications

* Pron pump inhibitors

* metformin

* selective serotonin Reuptake inhibitors

* inhibitors of gastric acid

* Anti-inflammatory drugs

Although you might need to take these medicines due to certain medical conditions, you'll should take extra precautions to ensure that the bacteria in your gut and digestive tract are in good health.

What are the reasons why antibiotics can affect your gut Health?

Antibiotics are made to kill the bacteria that reside in your body. However they are not all made to distinguish between healthy bacteria as well as the harmful bacteria that are creating you to become sick. Some antibiotics be able to target a variety of bacteria, which includes the beneficial gut bacteria. Other antibiotics may target a specific type of bacteria, causing less disruption to the gut bacteria. While using antibiotics you could notice an rise in nausea, diarrhea vomiting, stomach discomfort. Women can also suffer from yeast infections when taking antibiotics. This is because of the change in the dynamics of gut bacteria. This is the reason the reason why it is suggested that antibiotics are taken along in conjunction with food so that the gut bacteria is able to digest other food items.

It is generally advised that when taking antibiotics or complete your treatment, you consume probiotics in order to replenish your gut's microbiota.

What is the relation Between and the Gut as well as the Immune System?

If the GI tract is weakened it can trigger an immune system that weakens. The digestive tract and immune system are mirrored in regards to health. If you have a gut that is healthy, you're much more likely to be able to maintain a healthy as well-oiled immune system. When your digestive system is not healthy is more likely to have issues with your immune system.

How do I know whether I'm suffering from a food Allergy or intolerance?

Food intolerances and food allergies are often referred to as digestive issues which arise from eating certain foods. But, they are completely distinct. Food allergies consequence of your immune system experiencing an adverse reaction to specific kinds of food. Food allergies are a sign of an allergic reaction. appear almost instantly and be mild or even life-threatening. Signs of a food allergy are:

* tingling or itching in the mouth

* Red pimple

The swelling may be in the tongue, face or the extremities

* Tightening of the throat, which makes the swallowing process difficult and making it harder to breathe.

* vomiting or severe nausea

* anaphylaxis (which is a serious illness that affects the entire body and requires medical attention immediately)

Food intolerances, on one side, are caused as the digestive system has difficulty to digest a specific food. Food intolerance symptoms are not immediately apparent, but they do show up after a short period after eating. The symptoms may be present for only a few hours or could cause digestive problems for several days. The most common symptoms of food intolerances include:

* abdominal discomfort

* Bloating

* extra gas

* changes in the frequency of bowel movements or frequency

* skin irritations, rashes or skin rashes

What are the best supplements to help maintain a healthy Gut?

If you're eating a healthy, balanced diet with lots of plants supplementation isn't necessarily necessary. If you are struggling with digestive issues or think your diet isn't sufficient in nutrients as it should be, or are undergoing a major surgical or illness There are a few supplements to think about.

* prebiotics

* probiotics

* Essential fat acids

* digestive enzymes

* zinc

* Symbiotic (these are the supplements that possess both prebiotic and probiotic properties)

If you are a strict adherent to vegetarianism, your digestive system may also benefit from L Glutamine supplements. It can be an amino acid that is commonly digestible by eating foods such as eggs, red meat and beans, as well as other green vegetables. Because it is an amino acid, it aids the body to make protein blocks. For the gut, it could assist in providing energy to cells that reside inside the small intestines. It can also help repair damage to the intestine, and aid in the regulation of the inflammatory system.

There are other supplements that can aid in soothing and heal the digestive tract. Deglycyrrhizinated Licorice (DGL) as well as aloe vera as well as marshmallow root, are few examples of relaxing supplements. They have mucilage-like properties which will expand when combined with liquids. After digestion, these supplements assist in repairing the mucous membrane of the intestinal. They also help regulate the inflammatory response system.

Can Probiotics Help With Weight Loss?

Gut bacteria do have a significant impact on weight. The diversity of the gut microbiota can help to keep weight off and is the reason the reason many people think that once they start using probiotics, they'll notice significant weight reduction. Although probiotics can help replenish the gut microbiome however, they might not provide enough variety to help with weight loss.

It is important to modify your diet before you after that, add supplements. Your diet (as mentioned in chapter 6) should include many different plants-based foods. A balanced and healthy diet should concentrate on protein leanness, healthy fats and complex carbohydrates or high-fiber. A well-balanced diet can help beneficial bacteria flourish while helping to promote the growth of many of of bacteria.

Can you have too much of a good Quality Probiotics?

Probiotics are thought to be safe to consume in moderation, and although you may be tempted to add more of them to boost your the health of your gut, taking too many can cause negative side effects like:

Gas and bloating Gas and bloating occur in tandem because of the excessive gas being released by gut bacteria. Since the bacteria consume probiotics, they release gas that generally is not a problem since the average person could be expected to transmit gas as many as to 20 times per day. This could increase dramatically in the event that you take excessive probiotics. When there is an excess of gas in the body , it may cause you to feel uncomfortable and constipated. You might even notice your abdomen or stomach appears to be swollen and tight. The combination of excessive gas and bloating could make you feel more discomfort , or even pain.

Diarrrhea: If use too many probiotics, you could cause inflammation in your stomach. This can cause stool to become excessively watery, and you may experience more urgency to go to the bathroom. Diarrrhea isn't a problem when it lasts only one or two days. However when it continues to last for longer, it could suggest more serious health issues.

• Abdominal pain: These issues usually are accompanied by abdominal discomfort. The consumption of too many probiotics may result in intense pains, cramps and tightness around the stomach region.

www.ingramcontent.com/pod-product-compliance
Lightning Source LLC
Chambersburg PA
CBHW062140020426
42335CB00013B/1280